The HEALTHY
probiotic
Diet

Skyhorse Publishing books may be purchased in bulk at special discounts for sales promotion, corporate gifts, fund-raising, or educational purposes. Special editions can also be created to specifications. For details, contact the Special Sales Department, Skyhorse Publishing, 307 West 36th Street, 11th Floor, New York, NY 10018 or info@skyhorsepublishing.com.

Skyhorse® and Skyhorse Publishing® are registered trademarks of Skyhorse Publishing, Inc.®, a Delaware corporation.

www.skyhorsepublishing.com

10 9 8 7 6 5 4 3 2

Library of Congress Cataloging-in-Publication Data is available on file.

ISBN: 978-1-62914-202-9

Printed in the United States of America

Neither Skyhorse Publishing nor the author assume any liability for any health issues, including sickness, injury, or death, that arise from improper handling of probiotic cultures or the use or misuse of any of the instructions in this book. Brewing probiotic beverages requires patience and attention to detail. Always use caution and common sense when working with any fermented food or drink product.

The HEALTHY probiotic Diet

More Than 50 Recipes for Improved Digestion, Immunity, and Skin Health

R. J. RUPPENTHAL

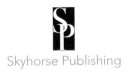

Skyhorse Publishing

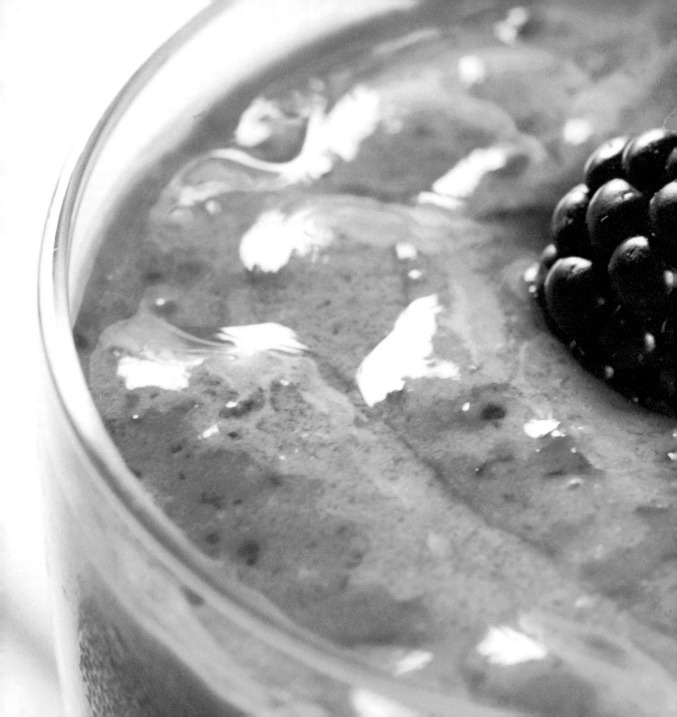

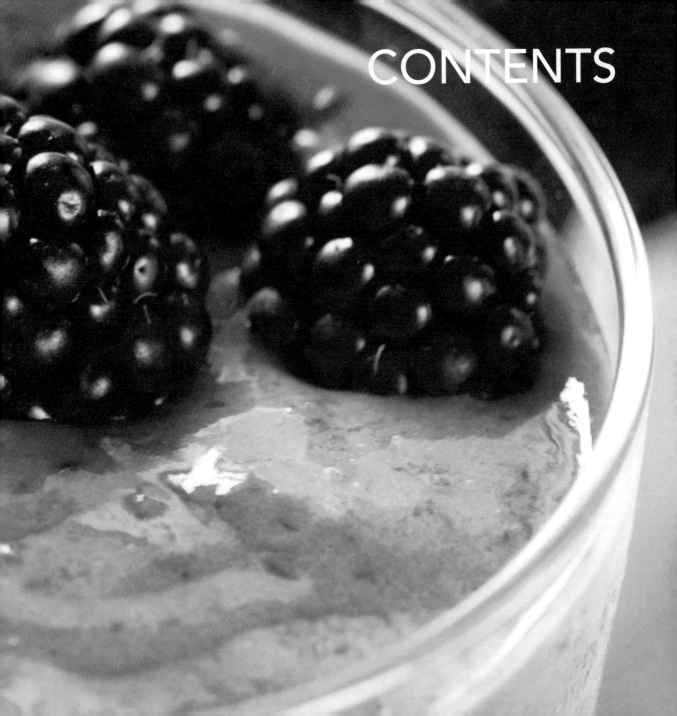

CONTENTS

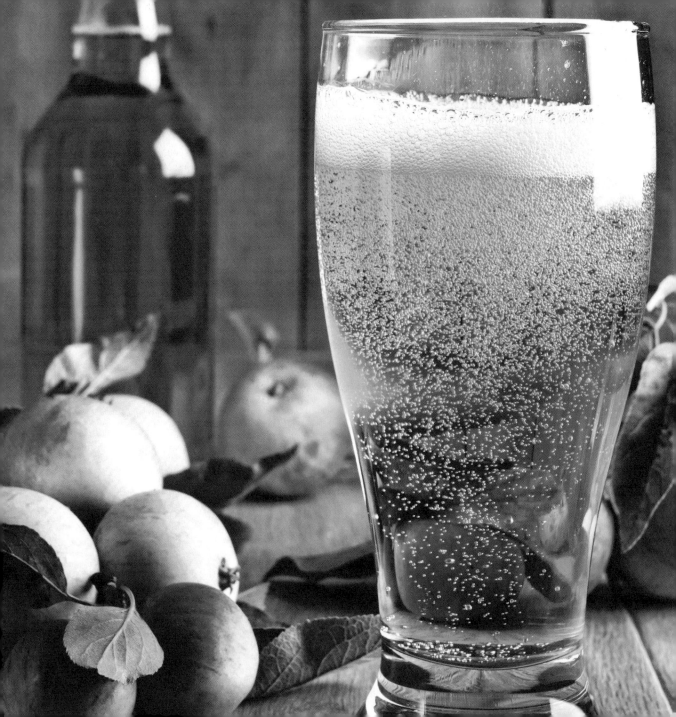

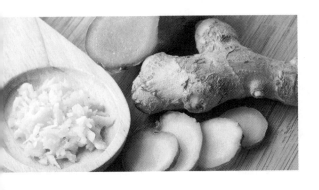
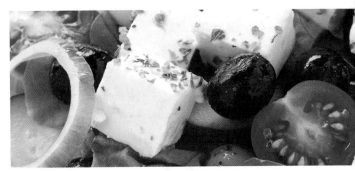

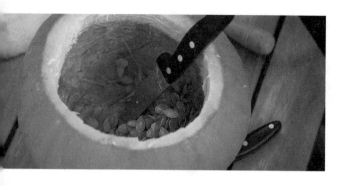
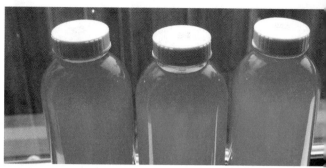

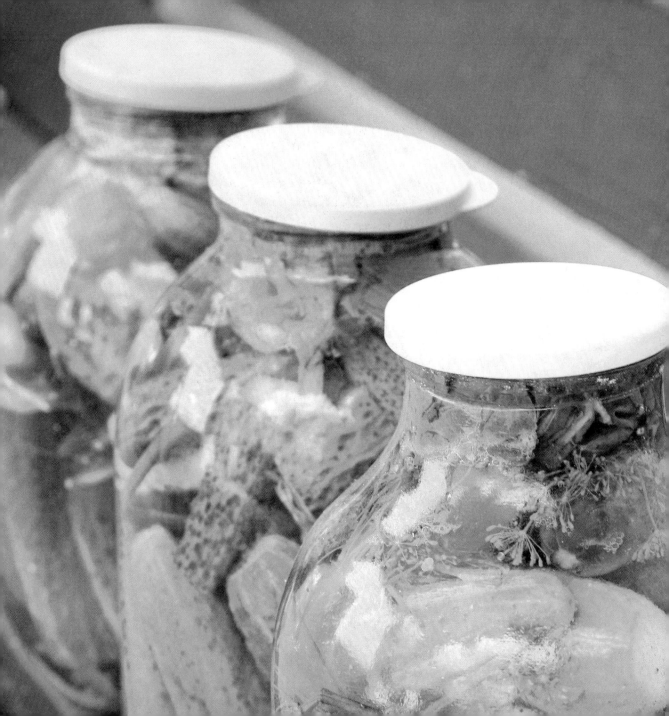

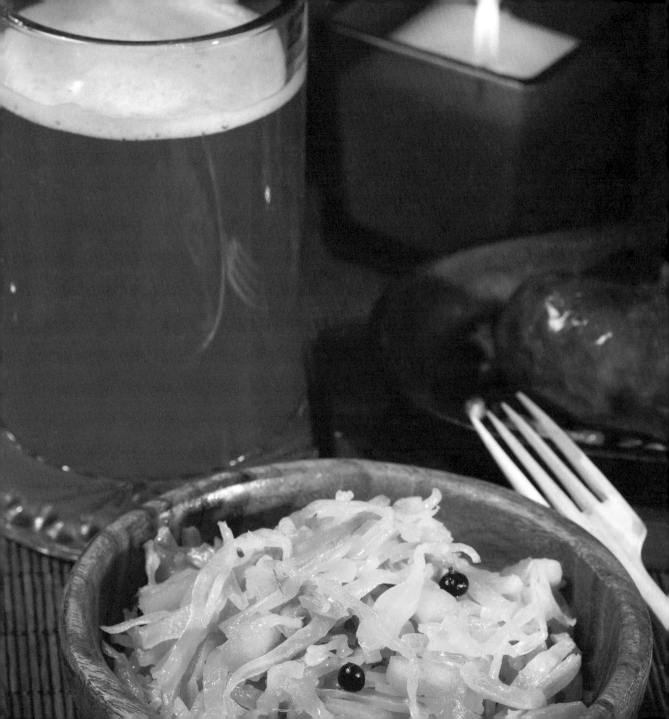

Chapter 1
The Basics of Probiotic Fermentation

In recent decades, a growing body of medical and nutritional research has confirmed that *probiotics are good for you.* People who take probiotics often experience better digestion, skin health, nutrient absorption, and immune system function, among other benefits. A healthy human body contains several pounds of bacteria and other microorganisms in its digestive tract. There, they help digest food that the body couldn't handle otherwise, produce beneficial enzymes and other compounds, and serve as a defense against unhealthy pathogenic organisms.

Scientists have demonstrated that certain species of bacteria and yeasts have a beneficial effect on the body. When people ingest these beneficial organisms, the populations of good bacteria seem to flourish. Meanwhile, the bad ones are kept in check and are not allowed to gain a foothold. These beneficial organisms have become known as probiotics. Good probiotics are particularly prevalent in lacto-fermented foods and drinks.

It stands to reason that if we want to stay healthy, we should include plenty of probiotics in our food. We can do this on an everyday basis by consuming lots of raw fruits and vegetables. Raw milk also contains some of these same organisms. But with today's highly refined and cooked diet, not to mention the pesticides on store-bought produce, it is difficult to ensure that we are getting the same probiotic effect as our bodies are built to expect.

Enter fermented foods and drinks, which can contain millions, billions, or even trillions of probiotics per serving. This makes them a much more concentrated source than the occurring bacteria in your average salad. Furthermore, a spoonful or two of fermented vegetables can contain more probiotic organisms than a whole jar of probiotic supplements from a health food store. As always, if you are suffering from a particular health condition, then it is always best to consult a physician or qualified natural health practitioner to make sure that probiotics are an advisable course of action. Generally, the risks and side effects are few to none.

When most people hear the word "fermentation," they think of wine, beer, and other alcoholic drinks. I enjoy the occasional drink myself, but alcoholic beverages are not included in this book because they are not probiotic. The only "beer" in this book is Ginger Beer, which is made using the original mother culture known as the ginger beer plant. It is only mildly (probably less than 1 percent) alcoholic.

Most alcoholic drinks are made with special yeast, which ferments the brew and leaves alcohol as a by-product. If they are not killed off earlier, then it is unlikely that any probiotic organisms would survive the aging of wine. Beer has a better chance of being probiotic, but the yeast generally crowds out any probiotic organisms, while hops is used both as a flavoring agent and a natural antibiotic.

This book covers probiotic cultures that can include beneficial lactobacteria, yeasts, and aceto acid bacteria. The best probiotic cultures contain several species of beneficial microorganisms living in balance. Probiotic beverages can contain small quantities (usually much less than 1 percent) of alcohol. But assuming that the yeast does not dominate a culture, the level of alcohol should remain much lower. This is because other bacteria can digest the alcohol and convert it to other substances, such as vinegary acetic acid.

My main interest in writing this book is to help you discover live cultured foods with a diverse array of probiotics. Therefore, the book does not include foods or drinks that only use fermentation at an early stage of preparation to create a sour flavor. If the rest of the process kills off this culture, then it may still be a great food or drink, but it isn't a useful probiotic anymore. Wine and beer are examples. People also use probiotic starter cultures to flavor cheese, but many kinds of cheese (not the ones in this book) are heated again to stop this fermentation. Sourdough bread starter is one more example: it can contain natural yeasts and bacteria, but these surely do not survive the oven. And ditto with Ethiopian injera or South Indian dosas, both of which are made from fermented grain or lentil flour that is cooked into sourdough crepes.

I eat my share of baked sourdough bread with pasteurized cheese, plus the occasional beer or wine. I am not 100 percent devoted to raw foods. But because this is a probiotic book, it stays true to the items that really deliver an honest probiotic benefit. In addition, many of the recipes here involve combining strong probiotic foods (such as yogurt and sauerkraut) with other ingredients to create a salad, dip, parfait, or other dish that remains high in probiotic power. Theoretically, you can add probiotic cultures this way to any food just before you eat it!

There are some wonderful cultured soy foods, such as miso (from Japan) and tempeh (from Indonesia). Unfortunately, I have not included them in this book because, so far, the scientific research on these foods has not shown that they are probiotic. Each one contains just a single species of fungus, not any probiotic bacteria, and research results have been mixed about their probiotic effects. As with wine, beer, or sourdough bread, simply being fermented does not make something probiotic. I will keep eating miso and tempeh, which no doubt have other health benefits, but they do not belong in a probiotic book.

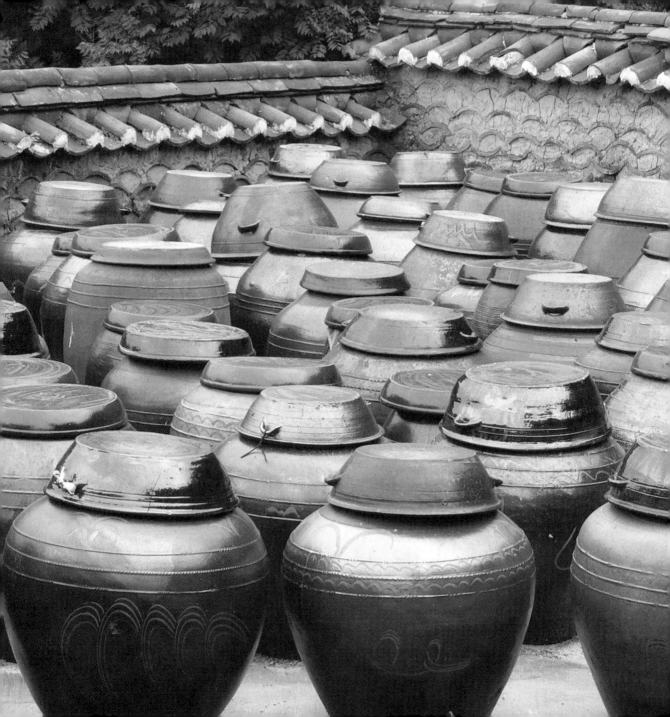

Probiotic Methods

All your pots, pans, jars, and utensils should be sterilized before you start fermenting. Pouring boiling water over them should do the trick. Sterilization will ensure you start with a clean slate of organisms and will help eliminate the chance of any contamination. Of course, some fermenters prefer to allow wild yeasts and naturally present bacteria to do their job. This is fine, since these naturally present organisms can ferment your foods and drinks just fine without you adding any cultures. However, wouldn't you rather culture the good guys that are on your fruits and vegetables, rather than whatever is on your equipment? The latter has more potential for mold, E. coli, and whatever is on the dog or cat hair floating around in your house. Sterilize first, and then, if you wish, you can ferment without adding any additional culture.

If you choose to add probiotic cultures, there are *three major ways* to create probiotic foods and drinks. The first is to place the food or drink in contact with a piece of permanent mother culture, such as kefir grains or kombucha mushrooms (they're not really grains or mushrooms, but those are the names often used to describe them). The probiotic organisms from this culture then colonize and ferment the food or drink.

The second way to inoculate food or drink with probiotics is to add to it some cultured material. This could be a spoonful of old sauerkraut, a few ounces of yogurt, yogurt whey (the liquid), kefir, water kefir, kombucha, rejuvelac, or ginger beer. Really any food or drink in this book will work as a starter for any other, since all are teeming with probiotics. Of course, you may not want a spoonful of spicy kimchi in your soda, so there are some limits.

Finally, sometimes you need to use some last-minute trickery to make a food or drink probiotic. Some foods are not fermented or fermentable, and sometimes they really should be cooked first; still, you can make them very effective probiotic foods by adding in some last-minute cultures before eating or drinking them. Cheating? Perhaps, but it's really a matter of learning how to use probiotic foods and drinks to create other recipes. The fermented porridge called Kunu or Koko (from Nigeria and Ghana) is made this way, with a portion of the raw probiotic grains being reserved and added again after the liquid portion has been cooked and cooled. The folks who developed that traditional recipe knew how to harness the best of both worlds.

At other times, a late probiotic addition just seems like the best idea. Take guacamole, for instance. You can lactoferment mashed avocadoes, but the oil in them can spoil in a hurry and turn brown as it oxidizes. Fermented guac is an acquired taste and I think I'll leave it to the purists. You can have a much fresher-tasting avocado dip, which contains plenty of probiotics, if you add a scoop of yogurt or a little chopped sauerkraut.

And what about smoothies? You can culture some fruit and it will become sour in a day or two. This book includes two wonderful fermented fruit recipes: Apple Chutney and Thanksgiving Cranberry-Orange Relish. Blend these into smoothies and you are sure to have more of a sour than sweet taste. Nothing wrong with this if you like it, but most people prefer sweeter smoothies. Instead, blend some fresh or frozen fruit along with some yogurt, kefir, kombucha, water kefir, or other probiotic drink. You will get the full probiotic benefit, plus the sweet flavors of fresh fruit.

As these examples illustrate, mixing in some probiotics at the last minute can be a great strategy. It is the quickest, easiest way to get more probiotics. Also, rather than fermenting half a dozen different dishes at one time, just ferment one or two (such as yogurt and kombucha). Using small amounts of these, you can make many other recipes, adding a great deal more probiotics to your diet without adding much to your workload.

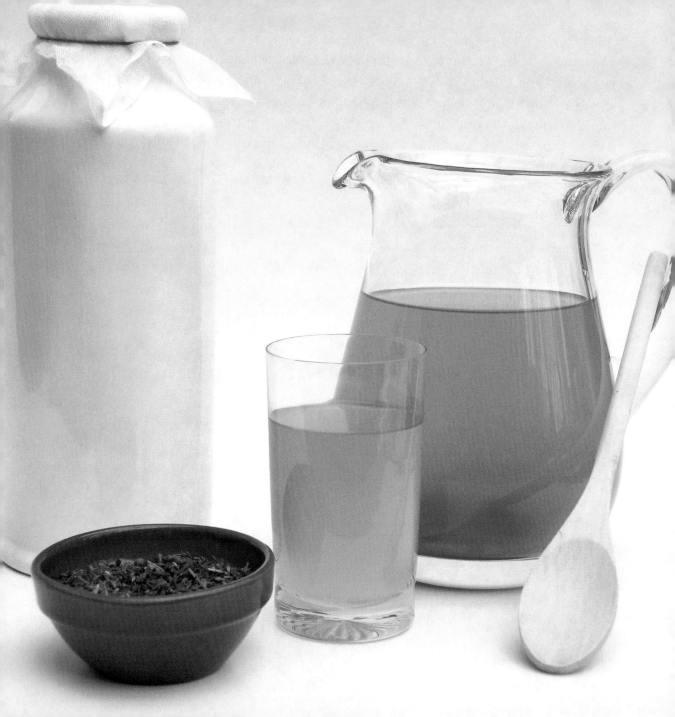

Chapter 2
Proper Equipment for Home Fermentation

Let's spend a moment discussing equipment and needs. To prepare most of the foods and drinks in this book, you will need many of the same basic containers and utensils. Because metal bowls and utensils can (theoretically) transmit small electrical charges that harm probiotic organisms, most fermenters prefer to use jars, containers, crocks, and utensils made of glass, BPA-free plastic, stone, silicon, and wood. For other recipes, you will need some standard kitchen items, such as a knife, cutting board, grater, mixing bowls, measuring cups and spoons, and pots and pans.

Here is a brief rundown of the more specialized items that are useful for preparing fermented foods and drinks. One worthy investment is a large plastic strainer with tight mesh. You can use this to strain cheese or Greek-style yogurt. Also, you can use it to recover large cultures from drinks, such as kombucha mushrooms, kefir grains, and tibicos. If you only have a plastic colander with larger holes, then another option is to line this with cheesecloth to make a good, tight strainer. Alternatively, you can use tight mesh straining bags, which are available in some health food stores and from online cheese-making supply stores.

To ferment probiotic foods, you can use almost any nonmetallic container. Traditionally, people from Germany to Korea make sauerkraut and kimchi in stone or earthenware crocks and pots. Many home fermenters use glass jars or BPA-free plastic containers to make these foods. On a smaller scale, you can prepare yogurt or dairy kefir using one or more cups, containers, bowls, or jars.

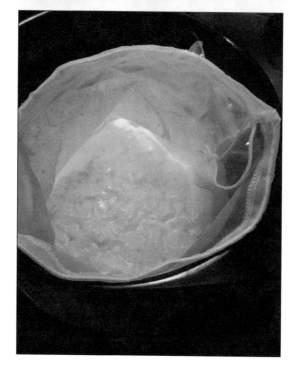

If you wish, for pickling, krauting, and other longer-term food fermentation projects, you can use the same type of air locks (also called pressure locks or water locks) that are used for making beer or cider. There are a couple of website resources listed in the appendix that sell pickling jars or lids that have air locks. These allow carbon dioxide to escape during fermentation while sealing the food from any outside contamination of mold, dust, insects, and debris.

Wooden spoons, plastic spoons, and silicon spatulas are three nonmetallic utensils that are particularly useful for stirring and moving fermented foods. If you plan to make any of the cheeses in this book, you will need extra equipment, including a large strainer, cheesecloth or straining bags, a cheese thermometer, and (for aged cheeses) a cheese mould and weight. All of these items are available at many health food stores and online at cheese-making supply stores.

To make water kefir, kombucha, and fermented cider, you will need a large jar or container. A beverage dispenser or water dispenser from one gallon to five gallons in size can work quite well for kombucha. If your dispenser has a valve and spout on the bottom, this usually will not get clogged by the kombucha SCOBY (symbiotic colony of bacteria and yeast, which generally sits near the top of the liquid), but kefir grains and any other items you add (like chopped ginger) can get stuck in it. To prevent this, consider putting these ingredients in a cloth bag and submerging it in the liquid.

To make sodas, you also will need some bottles. Any reused glass or plastic soda bottles can work well if they have reliable lids. Some home fermenters prefer using the traditional-looking glass soda bottles with clasp tops, which are available online and from home-brewing supply stores. Also, many of the soda recipes include recipes for flavoring syrups that involve cooking in a small pot or pan.

The most important piece of equipment for smoothies, parfaits, and frozen drinks is a good blender. Smoothies are only smooth if your blender can purée chunks of fruit. For frozen smoothies, your blender must be able to slush up any frozen fruit or ice you choose to add. You may prefer to use a food processor, which also can work well for many smoothies. The best smoothie blender I have ever used is the Ninja™, which is basically a high-powered blender with a food processor blade. If you can afford a real commercial blender, then go for it, but for me the Ninja was the next best thing and was worth every penny of the $100 or so that it cost.

Finally, you will need to obtain the cultures to ferment your food. With yogurt, buttermilk, sauerkraut, and natural pickles, this is a simple matter of buying some in the store and using a small bit of its culture to inoculate your homemade batch. With others, such as kefir, water kefir (tibicos), kombucha, and ginger beer, you

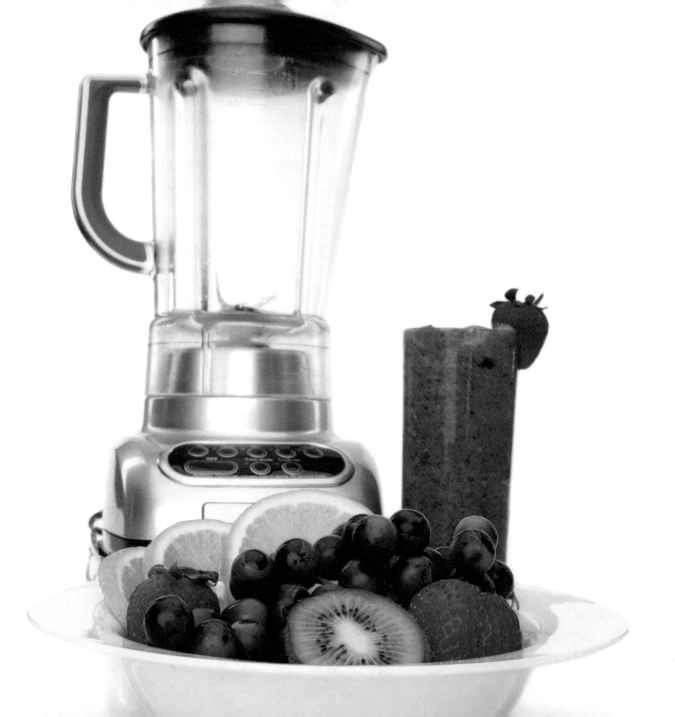

must obtain the culture from someone else who has it. Though it is possible to grow your own kombucha mushroom from store-bought kombucha, I recommend buying this culture the first time.

If you do not know anyone who ferments with these cultures, you can buy some online to get started. Please check the appendix at the end of this book, it contains a list of several great websites that sell reliable cultures.

You may need additional items to make certain foods and drinks in this book; but these are the main tools of fermentation. As other items are needed, they are noted in the recipes.

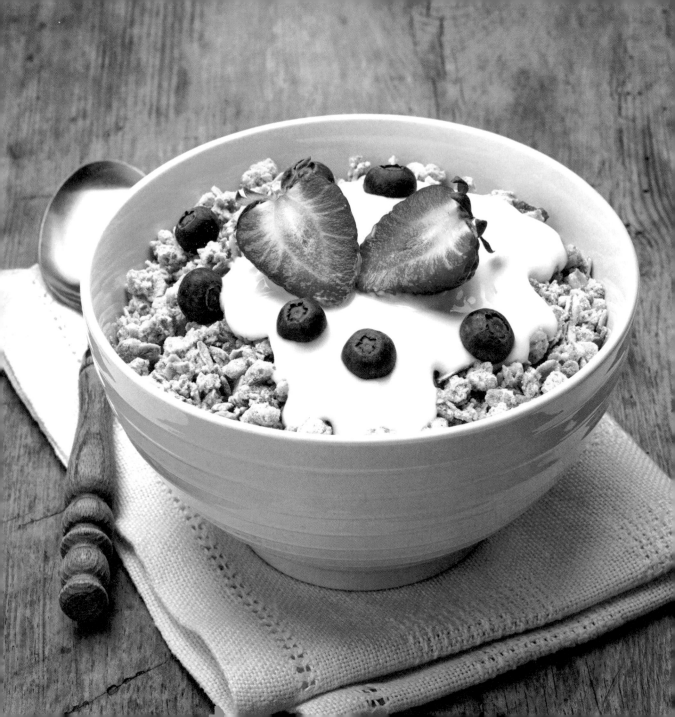

Chapter 3
How This Book Works

The recipes in this book are designed to be very simple. The only exception is the gouda cheese recipe, which is probably the most complex one I have included (yet it is still quite achievable). Most recipes in this book use yogurt, kefir, water kefir, kombucha, cider, pickles, or sauerkraut as base ingredients. For example, the Blackberry Smoothie recipe calls for yogurt or kefir, while the Chai Spiced Soda recipe uses a base of kombucha, cider, or water kefir. For the solid-foods recipes, you can chop up some natural pickles to make the Egg Salad probiotic, while the Burmese Green Tea Salad recipe incorporates sauerkraut, and you can make a delicious Kimchi Noodles dish using kimchi.

On the surface, using these fermented foods as base ingredients would seem to lengthen the time needed to make any of the other recipes. Instead, I am hoping that using yogurt and sauerkraut in your recipes will save you time. Here's why: As you develop a culture of fermentation in your own household (sorry for the pun), I am hoping that you will have ready access to the basics, such as yogurt, kombucha, natural pickles, and/or sauerkraut. Once you make a batch of sauerkraut, you can keep eating it for months, so I am not asking you to make more every time you want to prepare another recipe.

Yogurt and kefir do not last as long as sauerkraut, but they literally take just minutes to make, and therefore it is pretty easy to have all the yogurt or kefir you need by whipping up a quick batch every week. Once you have yogurt or kefir, making smoothies is just a matter of doing some blending.

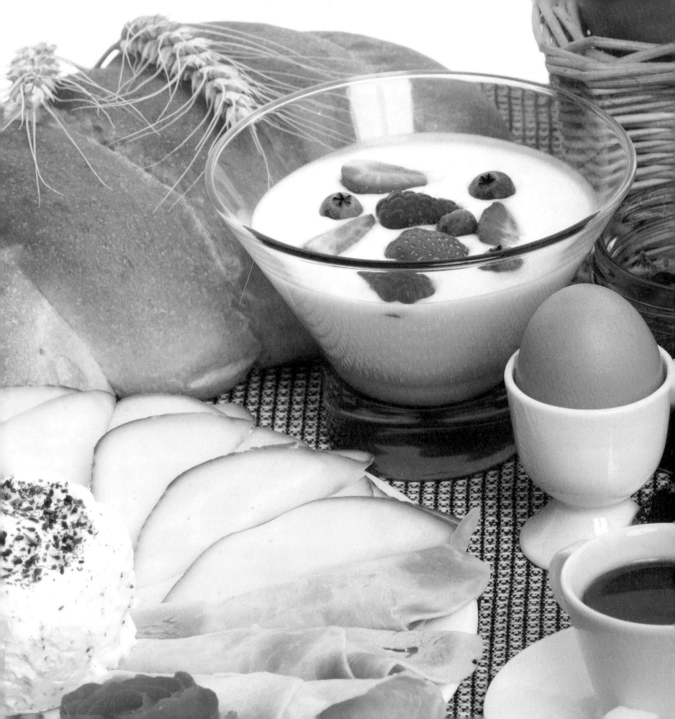

A number of the recipes call for direct fermentation. For example, the Garlic Mustard, Hummus, and Chocolate Coconut Pudding recipes call for the finished product to be cultured first and then fermented for an additional period. This final step is always optional, since the foods already contain a probiotic starter culture (such as yogurt water, called whey). But the additional fermentation stage radically increases the probiotic content of your foods and adds an additional layer of sour flavor to the taste.

Several recipes in this book contain a double- or triple-whammy of probiotics. The Dolmas recipe, for example, requires first fermenting some grape leaves, then stuffing them with an herbed rice filling accented by yogurt, and finally letting the wrapped dish ferment for an additional period. *Did I mention you will be getting your probiotics? Oh yes!*

When it comes to fermenting vegetables and fruits, I will give you a choice of cultures. The easiest thing to do is to culture your fermentation with a spoonful or two of yogurt whey, water kefir, kombucha, or other fermented food or drink. In addition, it is quite possible to ferment fruits and vegetables using naturally present yeasts and lactobacteria. Yes, they really are in the air, on your produce, and on your kitchen utensils, and most of them are very good for you.

With this sort of "wild fermentation," which was popularized by Sandor Katz in his terrific book by that name, there is always a small potential of risk. The majority of the time, wild fermentation works very well, and you end up with a nicely fermented product with a healthy blend of organisms. With the fermented fruit and veggie dishes, you generally are using a salt brine, so this encourages beneficial lactobacteria while making it pretty difficult for others (like mold or anaerobic bacteria) to colonize your food. Wild fermentation certainly is a solid option, which many people use for foods like sauerkraut and kimchi. Just omit the culture ingredient in any of the fermented vegetable and fruit recipes in this book, and you should be fine.

However, some folks are not comfortable with trusting some unknown organisms to culture their food. If you are in the camp that would rather control your culture, then do not fear, since these recipes are designed for you. That is why yogurt whey, kombucha, water kefir, or another fermented culture are ingredients in each of these recipes. These cultures will dominate and prevent any molds or other organisms from forming, so adding them to your foods provides a very safe way to culture a fermented dish.

Still, there are some potential issues with using yogurt whey, water kefir, or kombucha to culture vegetables and fruits. First, kombucha and the tibicos cultures used to make water kefir both contain yeasts (and usually aceto acid bacteria as well). There is nothing wrong with these, which appear to be very healthy and probiotic. However, moving them to a base of vegetables and asking them to culture the vegetables can throw their balance out of whack. Particularly with a longer ferment (which is needed with kombucha culture, especially), one part of the culture can become dominant. If the yeast predominates, as it often does when you leave something a little too long using kombucha or kefir grain cultures, then your food will start tasting kind of yeasty. It is still quite edible, but less tasty, unless you really have a thing for ale and sourdough bread.

The second issue is as follows: the (definitely beneficial) probiotic organisms that culture foods and drinks such as yogurt and kombucha are not the same ones that naturally occur on vegetables and fruits. Yogurt bacteria, for example, have been chosen for their ability to culture and metabolize lactose. Put them on some cabbage or apples and there's no lactose there. Yes, there are other sugars in plants, and yes, the lactobacteria will be able to metabolize them. They will do a fine job of culturing veggies and fruits.

But limiting the cultures you eat to *L. acidophilus* and its buddies means that you are not getting significant amounts of the organisms naturally present on fruits and vegetables. These are primarily soil-based organisms with a wider cast of characters, including a number of different *Bifidobacteria*. Research has shown that strains do matter, and that a diversity of different organisms seems to promote better digestive and immune system health. Our bodies are developed to eat more raw vegetables and fruits than most of us eat today. At one time, our ancestors probably ingested a good deal more of these soil-based organisms that are naturally found on produce. Is it important for our bodies' health to eat more of these also?

If so, then here is a good way for you to obtain some natural vegetable culture that you can keep on using. Before you make your first batch of fermented foods, buy a batch of high-quality sauerkraut at a health food store and save some of the juice as your first culture. Then you can keep using a little juice from your last ferment every time you need to make another one. Alternatively, you can buy a vegetable culture online and start with this. Either way, if you make fermentation an ongoing habit, then you may never need to buy another culture again. It's a one-time gift to yourself that will keep on giving.

Raw Diets

A raw diet refers to the presence of active enzymes and live food compounds in the fermented foods you create. Probiotic foods must be raw since cooking kills the beneficial microorganisms that make them probiotic. Every recipe in this book helps you make foods and drinks that are rich with raw probiotics by the time you eat or drink them.

In addition, most recipes in this book use raw base ingredients. However, I allow cooking for grains and beans because many people are accustomed to eating them this way. Bean and grain recipes in this book use *cooked* beans and grains. They will still be cultured with probiotics before you eat them, so will have plenty of enzymes. But if you are adept at soaking and sprouting your own grains and beans, and your body is able to digest these in serious quantities, then feel free to go 100 percent raw and use these instead in your probiotic recipes. I enjoy eating sprouted grains and beans (I even wrote a book on sprouting), but I only eat these as snacks or salad sprinklings; my body cannot handle them in large portions. Hats off to the hard-core raw foodies, but I'm with the 99 percent who cook some of their food.

Milk Issues and CRASH Substitutions

Many people do not have access to raw milk, while others are sensitive to lactose and therefore do not consume dairy products. For the yogurt, kefir, cheese, smoothie, and other dairy-related items in this book, you are welcome to use either pasteurized or raw milk. Frankly, I would suggest pasteurized, just because raw milk comes with an uncertain blend of bacteria. Some of them are very good for you and you may want to culture them, but there also may be a few undesirables in there. By beginning with pasteurized milk, you have a clean slate to culture milk with beneficial probiotic cultures, far more than raw milk contains.

Please *do not* use ultra-pasteurized milk (or "U.P.") milk to make probiotic foods. U.P. milk has been heated to an unnaturally hot temperature. This changes the chemical structure of milk to make it shelf stable. Because the composition of the food has changed, lactobacteria cannot culture it very well. Regular pasteurized milk is fine.

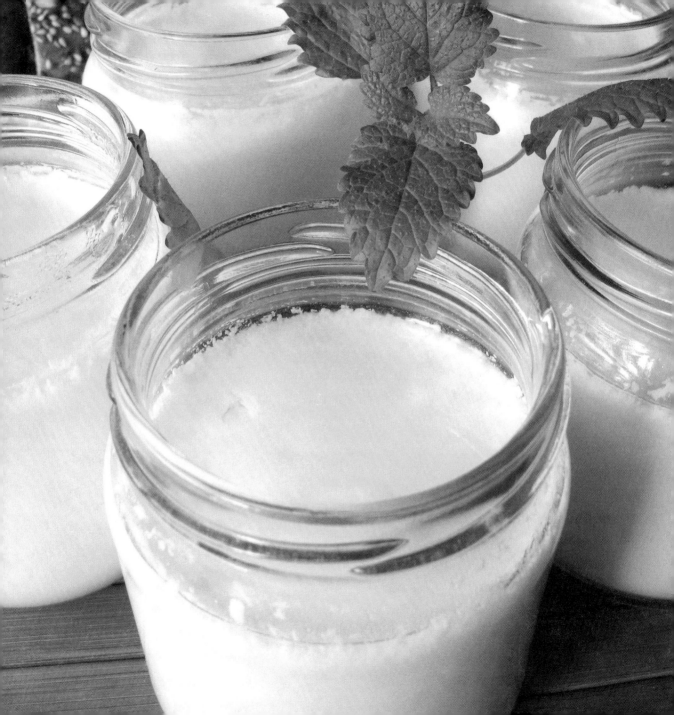

If you are lactose intolerant ("allergic to dairy"), then you are welcome to substitute with nondairy "milks." In the recipes in this book (mostly the smoothie ones), I label these other milks as "CRASH alternatives." CRASH is an acronym for coconut, rice, almond, soy, and hemp milks. CRASH has no overt or hidden meaning. I simply started using it as shorthand in the recipes and it caught on. However, flaxseed milk is being sold in stores also, and I'm sure there are other alternative dairy beverages, so I may need to come up with a new term soon!

If you are making yogurt or kefir, then culturing high protein milks like soy can take a little longer, but it works. I suggest adding a small quantity of sugar or maple syrup at first to get the good bacteria off to a faster start.

However, most people who are lactose intolerant are able to eat good quality yogurt, kefir, and cheese. There are two reasons for this. First, the lactobacteria (and yeasts in kefir) digest most of the lactose. In fact, a few brands of yogurt, kefir, and cheese are marketed as being 100 percent lactose-free. Second, the beneficial organisms in these fermented milks also produce lactase, which is the enzyme that digests lactose.

If you are lactose intolerant, then most likely your body is not "allergic" to milk. It simply cannot produce the lactase enzyme to digest it. So even if the yogurt or kefir you like is not 100 percent lactose-free, the lactase in it will enable most people to digest any lactose that remains. If you have any specific medical condition, then check with a physician, but experiment if you are able to do so and you may well find that cultured fermentation solves the problem.

Sweet / Sour Variations

There is one other variable in many of this book's recipes. When you make your own yogurt or kombucha, you may like it really sour, while someone else prefers it milder. You may stop your yogurt fermentation after 6–8 hours because you like it creamy and mild, while your neighbor lets it go for 10 hours for a fully sour flavor. You may stop your kombucha culture and refrigerate it a day or two earlier than someone else does.

Many recipes in this book build upon these basic fermented foods and drinks. A smoothie or salad dressing recipe may incorporate yogurt. A homemade soda recipe may use kombucha. And since your kombucha and someone else's may be different, that creates the possibility of some serious variation in the recipes as well.

The main potential variation is with sourness. And if something is really sour, it may be inherently less sweet. So feel free to adjust sourness and sweetness as you wish in each recipe. Add more sour flavor with additional yogurt, kefir, water kefir, kombucha, or lemon juice. Add more sweetness with sugar, maple syrup, honey, or another natural sweetener substitute.

Finally, the fermented vegetable recipes can come out pretty salty. Using a certain level of saltiness helps ensure a clean fermentation using lactobacteria. But if a recipe is too salty for you, feel free to cut back on the salt, or add a little more of the bulky ingredients to compensate.

Using Water, Sugar, and Salt Properly

Water: If there is one prohibited ingredient in this book, it is chlorinated water. The chlorine is designed to kill off microorganisms, including the good ones (oops) you need to culture your food. So please do not add chlorinated water to your recipes if you want to keep them probiotic; it is the same as adding bleach to your food and drinks. If your tap water is chlorinated, then either filter it or use bottled water to make these cultured foods and drinks. By the way, you shouldn't drink your water without filtering it, either, since your body's digestive system will take a hit of chlorine each time you do.

Sugar: As with salt, most probiotic recipes are best when you use a whole, balanced sugar. Evaporated cane sugar is great, brown sugar is fine, and maple syrup does a good job also. Each of these contains minerals and whole food components in addition to the sweet part. White sugar just has the sweet part with the rest of the goodness removed. Unless a recipe mentions otherwise, please use a whole sugar. Kombucha is the only exception I can think of in which white sugar is better, and this is because it balances particularly well with the tea (already a whole food) to feed the organisms in the culture. In most recipes that call for sugar as a sweetener, you can substitute with honey, xylitol, agave, apple juice, or another natural substance. But when you are specifically feeding a probiotic fermentation, such as with water kefir grains, a whole sugar is best.

Sea Salt: You will notice that the recipes generally call for sea salt rather than just plain old table salt. Iodized salt actually is a very imbalanced combination of minerals. Yes, our bodies need iodine, but they also need all the other trace elements that are missing from table salt. Sea salt contains these trace minerals in appropriate proportions for both the human body and for the microorganisms that we need to culture our probiotic foods. Please use sea salt or any other whole salt, such as Celtic salt, grey salt, Real Salt™, Himalayan pink salt, and the like. All of these are basically sea salt with some regional differences in the mineral deposits.

Warning: Contents Under Pressure

Be very careful when using glass and breakable vessels when fermenting foods and drinks. Fermentation increases the pressure and expands the space within these containers. With any active fermentation there is always a small possibility that a container will crack or pop. This has never happened to me, but I always recommend checking your cultures daily or even more frequently if possible. As the author of this book, I do not wish to promote any activity that leads to potential injuries.

Though some fermenters put tight lids on their fermenting foods, I always cover containers loosely to allow the CO_2 to escape. I often use a napkin or paper towel as a cover and place the lid on top of it, so that this material screens out most dust or mold spores floating in the air. The only exception to my loose covering is with ciders and the secondary fermentation of sodas. Plastic soda bottles are easier to check (just squeeze to determine the pressure level). If you use glass soda bottles, please keep a very close eye on tightly capped ones. Also, contents can spurt out if shaken, as you probably know if you are a consumer of store-bought kombucha, so please avoid shaking.

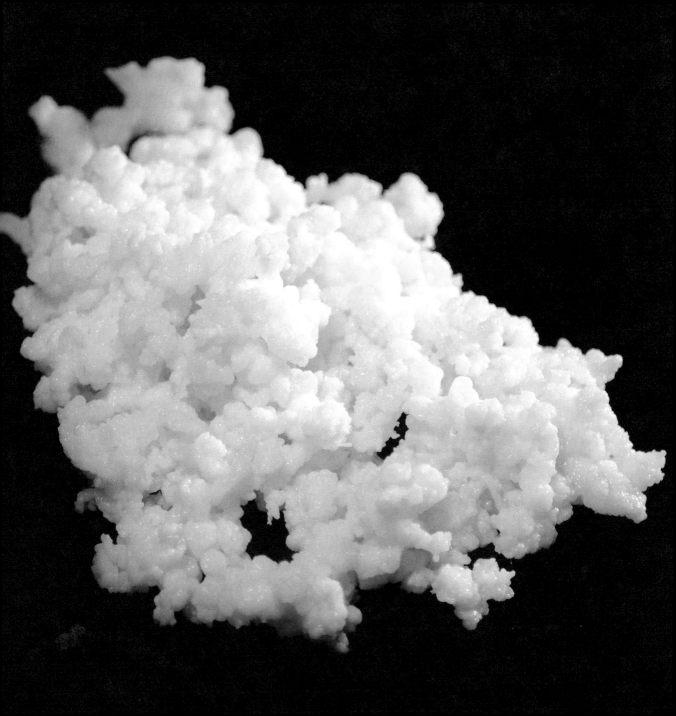

Chapter 4
SCOBYs: The Probiotic Mother Cultures

Yogurt cultures are nearly invisible. You start with either some cloudy milk or a powdered version of this. But authentic kefir, kombucha, and ginger beer are made with a permanent mother culture, which we will call a SCOBY. The term SCOBY stands for symbiotic community of bacteria and yeasts. A SCOBY is large enough that you can see it, handle it gently, and move it to wherever you need the culture.

Each SCOBY is an amazingly stable and diverse community of organisms. These bacteria and yeasts are the original probiotics of our ancestors, handed down for thousands of years from generation to generation. There are some variations between the different SCOBYs, but research has revealed that each kind tends to contain some of the same beneficial species of yeasts, lactobacteria, and aceto acid bacteria. Once you have a SCOBY, you can keep maintaining it indefinitely, as our ancestors have done. And you can use it to culture any food or drink in this book, plus many more.

To culture a drink, you simply put the proper SCOBY in it. In a matter of hours or days, your drink will ferment. You just need to include the proper ingredients and keep it in a still place until your probiotic drink is ready.

Each kind of SCOBY is accustomed to feeding on (and thereby fermenting) particular foods. For example, kombucha SCOBYs (known as "kombucha mushrooms" or "the kombucha mother") have been developed to ferment sweet tea. Brew some tea, add some sugar, and the kombucha cultures will thrive. Similarly, kefir grains (which resemble small milk curds) contain a high proportion of lactobacteria. Since these species can metabolize lactose, they are great for fermenting milk.

Water kefir grains are virtually identical to dairy kefir grains except that they normally appear translucent rather than white. Water kefir grains were developed to culture sugar water or juice. The lactobacteria can metabolize sucrose (table sugar), while the yeasts are well suited to breaking down the fructose in fruit juice. In both cases, simple sugars, which the organisms can eat as they ferment your drink, are left over. The ginger beer plant (or "ginger beer mother") is another SCOBY that has been developed to make naturally fermented ginger beer from water, sugar, and ginger.

You can use SCOBYs to culture solid food dishes also, from sauerkraut to cottage cheese. There are two options for this. First, you can put some of the SCOBY culture into whatever food you want to culture (such as putting kefir grains in some shredded cabbage to make sauerkraut). Second, you can simply pour off some cultured fluid from the SCOBY. For example, a few tablespoons of kombucha or water kefir contain enough of the starter culture to ferment any of the solid food dishes in this book. If you use fluid as a culture rather than the SCOBY itself, you probably will get a more uniform and even fermentation. Also, you will not have to go digging through your fermented food to find pieces of the SCOBY and pull them out again. But either method works fine.

To maintain your SCOBYs, you need to continue feeding them regularly. This basically consists of keeping them in a drink that includes whatever they like to eat (milk, sugar water, etc.). You need to keep adding more every few days. If you stop feeding them, they will die, and you will need to start again with a fresh SCOBY.

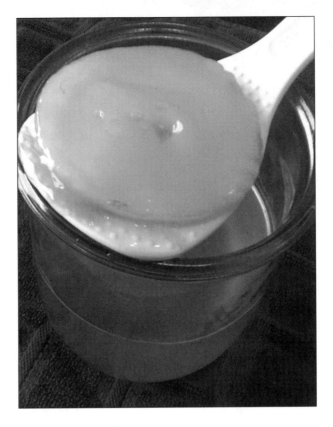

If you need to take a break from fermenting, you can store your kefir grains in the refrigerator in some milk/sugar water. This will ferment in the refrigerator, but quite slowly, as the organisms' metabolism slows way down in cool temperatures. You can store the SCOBY grains like this for up to two weeks at a time. If you need to store your culture longer, then change out the fluid and replace it with some more milk or sugar water. For kombucha SCOBYs, it is best not too refrigerate because the yeasts can go dormant and take a while to awaken later, which throws the culture out of balance. Just keep the mushroom going in a room-temperature drink, even if you do not plan to drink it. Kombucha drinks take a while to ferment anyway, so you probably can fit in a vacation for a week or two.

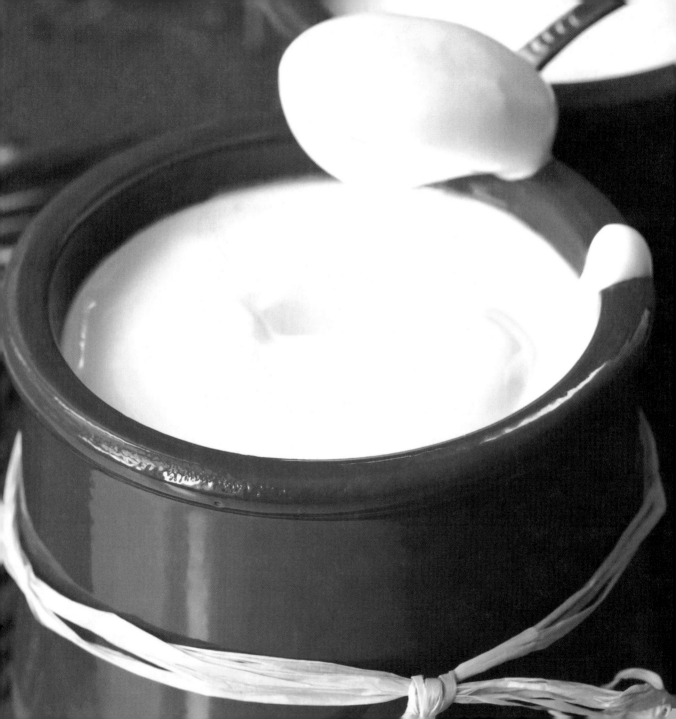

Chapter 5
Yogurt, Kefir, and Buttermilk

Yogurt, kefir, and buttermilk are fermented milk products that are simple to make at home. Yogurt is thickened milk that is cultured by several species of beneficial bacteria. It has a solid, pudding-like texture that people generally eat with a spoon. Buttermilk is a thickened but drinkable beverage that is cultured with a different set of bacteria than yogurt; the species that make up buttermilk culture are actually the same as those found in many cheese cultures. Kefir is a drinkable yogurt, which usually is cultured with a broader range of probiotic organisms that include both beneficial bacteria and yeasts.

Fermented milks have a long history, probably originating thousands of years ago in Central Asia. Experts have suggested that the first fermented milk came about when herders stored their goat or sheep milk in skin pouches. Bacteria and yeast that were naturally present began to metabolize the lactose in the milk, fermenting it into kefir or yogurt.

Over time, people selected the best cultures and continued to maintain them. Not only did they like the sour taste but they also found that fermenting milk was a great way to preserve it for a journey. Both yogurt and kefir came to be associated with health benefits from the probiotic bacteria and live food enzymes. These include improved digestion, better skin health, enhanced immunity, and better nutrient absorption.

Today, yogurt is a controlled culture that contains a few strains of friendly lactobacteria. Kefir remains slightly wilder and can contain both yeasts and bacteria. Somewhere in their history, the two related foods diverged and their cultures were refined separately. There are some regional variations in yogurt as well. People probably refined these cultures over time to suit their own climates and tastes.

Yogurt was well-known in both ancient Persia and India, where records suggest that its use goes back at least six thousand years. In the first century BC, Cleopatra famously took yogurt baths to keep her skin vibrant. The Roman author Pliny the Elder wrote that certain Nomadic tribes knew how to thicken milk into a substance with a pleasing acidic taste.

Traditionally, buttermilk was a by-product of making butter from cultured cream. Today, it is generally made by culturing milk with a particular blend of lactobacteria. Though buttermilk is not as popular as a probiotic, and its bacterial strains are not chosen for their probiotic qualities, it is a high-quality fermented drink with many of the same health benefits as its close cousins. If you prefer buttermilk to yogurt or kefir, then please feel free to make it and use it in any of the recipes (smoothies, for example) that call for yogurt or kefir.

True kefir is made from kefir grains, which are particles of the culture that look like wet popcorn or cottage cheese curds. These remarkably stable communities of microorganisms form kefir's mother culture, which has been handed down from generation to generation. Legend has it that the prophet Muhammad made a gift of kefir grains to the people of the Caucasus region, telling them to safeguard its secret. And safeguard it they did.

For centuries, the people living between the Black and Caspian seas kept their kefir grains a secret. Travelers on trade routes through the region, as well as on the main Silk Road, to the south, carried stories of kefir but were unable to obtain its recipe. Marco Polo tasted it and described kefir in the accounts of his travels. Yet for centuries thereafter, kefir making remained confined to the Caucasus.

By the early twentieth century, Russians in the north badly wanted the secret recipe. A large Russian dairy, backed by a physicians' group, hatched a plan to obtain some kefir grains. They sent a very beautiful woman as a spy to charm some kefir grains from a local prince of the Caucasus. However, the prince would not give them up. Instead, he kidnapped the woman as she left, intending to marry her. The Russian dairy mounted a rescue attempt to save her from marriage to the prince, who now had committed a crime under Russian law. When he was arrested, the Russians forced the prince to hand over some kefir grains. And thus, kefir conquered Russia, where it became a dietary staple. Today, the average Russian drinks 5.68 gallons (21.5 liters) of kefir per year. This works out to about two ounces (58 milliliters) per day.

We will cover the formal process of making yogurt, buttermilk, and kefir next. Just so you know, it is pretty simple. There are just two ingredients: the milk and the culture!

Yogurt

Yogurt is the simplest cultured food to make, so it's a great place to start. You need two ingredients: good quality milk and a source of yogurt culture. Organic or grass-fed milk is always best, but any milk will do. Make sure the milk has not been ultra-pasteurized, a process of heating it at high temperatures that changes its chemistry and makes it difficult to ferment. However, the milk should be pasteurized (as opposed to raw milk). Raw milk already can contain some bacterial cultures, which may interfere with your yogurt fermentation. Unless you have 100 percent faith in your source of raw milk, just use pasteurized milk to make yogurt.

There are two possible sources of yogurt culture, and I recommend the second one. Your first choice is to start with some powdered yogurt starter culture, which you can buy online or in a health food store. If you are using a dry, powdered starter, it is best to follow the directions on the package to make yogurt. Dry starter works quite well and is a portable option, but if you're using it frequently, dry starter becomes an expensive way to make yogurt. Another issue is that most dry starters are not strong enough to make multiple batches. In other words, you cannot save some of the yogurt from each batch to culture the next batch; after a batch or two, it loses strength.

A much easier and more affordable way to get started is to buy some good yogurt. If it's good, then it has plenty of live active cultures in it to ferment your milk. Check the label for the term "live cultures" or "active cultures" to make sure it is potent. Plain, sour yogurt makes the best starter, since flavored yogurts contain other ingredients and can impart an off-taste to the end product. This *will* give you a source of perpetual culture you can use again and again.

You will need about one-eighth to one-sixth as much yogurt starter as milk. So, for example, you can use one six-ounce (single serving) container of yogurt to culture enough milk to make 6–8 servings of yogurt. A higher proportion of yogurt starter will make for a faster fermentation.

Most yogurts in the store will list their bacterial cultures on the label. The majority of them use just a few cultures, most commonly *Lactobacillus acidophilus*, *Lactococcus thermophilus*, and *Lactobacillus bulgaricus.* But in recent years, researchers have taken a closer look at probiotics, and the results have proven that certain strains of bacteria offer health benefits. Today, more yogurt makers include these than ever before.

Some additional Lactobacillus cultures that now appear in yogurts include *L. casei, L. paracasei, L. reuteri, L. rhamnosus, L. plantarum*, and *Bifidobacterium*, though there are others as well. Each of these species has shown promise in providing immune system enhancement, improved digestion, and other health benefits. Therefore, if you can get some store-bought yogurt that includes one or more of these strains, it should make a healthy starter culture. In practice, not all species of friendly bacteria will culture well at the same temperature, and some probably are added after fermentation in these store-bought yogurts. But at least a broad spectrum of beneficial organisms is present with your starter, and hopefully a few of them will make it through to give you a broad range of beneficial organisms in your new cultured batch.

Buttermilk

The process of making buttermilk is the same as for yogurt. You just need to start with buttermilk cultures rather than yogurt cultures, because they are different. The best source of buttermilk cultures is buttermilk itself, so first you will need to buy some at the store that contains "live" or "active" cultures. While buttermilk uses the same bacteria as some cheese starters, do not attempt to use cheese cultures to make buttermilk. This is because the strains of bacteria and their ratios may be slightly different and you might not like the taste of what comes out.

Buttermilk cultures will grow just fine at room temperature. Start with a large container, bowl, or jar. Warm some milk to around room temperature or slightly warmer. Pour or scoop some buttermilk into the container/bowl/jar, then cover with the milk, stir it up, cover the container, and let it sit for 24–36 hours. For example, to make about a quart of buttermilk, heat one quart of milk to room temperature and combine it with a cup of buttermilk, then mix, cover, and let sit. Check it after 24 hours and let it go longer if you like sour buttermilk. Alternatively, you can make buttermilk in a large yogurt maker; just remember to check it before 24 hours because the warmer temperature can accelerate the fermentation.

Buttermilk doesn't get much love in this book. The recipes here are written with yogurt and kefir, rather than buttermilk, in mind. The cultures in yogurt and kefir are considered to be more probiotic, which is why I prefer them. Yet buttermilk contains some beneficial lactobacteria as well, and there is no doubt that these create a creamier flavor than the yogurt bacteria do. You have my permission to enjoy your homemade buttermilk and to substitute it for yogurt or kefir in this book's recipes!

Kefir

Stores are selling more kefirs and drinkable yogurts these days also. In fact, for marketing purposes, the term "kefir" basically means drinkable yogurt. Most "kefirs" you can buy in stores are just milk with yogurt cultures. Read the label and you'll see this "kefir" contains the same species of friendly bacteria found in yogurt. I love drinkable yogurt, but I would not call it kefir.

Real kefir should be made from kefir grains, which will give it a cultured blend of both beneficial bacteria and yeasts. Many experts believe that the cultures in kefir are stronger and better able to colonize a person's digestive tract than yogurt cultures. Having a healthy population of friendly microorganisms in your digestive system can help your body to properly digest.

Despite our preoccupation with hand sanitizers, antibiotics, and mouthwashes to kill as many microorganisms as possible, the average human body contains about three to five pounds of bacteria. Though these organisms are small, there are so many of them that bacteria cells in the human body outnumber the human cells by ten to one. Without friendly bacteria, we would experience a lot more digestive problems and diseases. If you want to stay healthy, one of the best things you can do is to encourage a healthy community of microorganisms to flourish in your digestive system. Kefir can help make this happen.

If someone you know uses kefir grains, you should be able to get a small amount from him or her. Just a tablespoon or two of kefir grains is enough for starters. You can purchase some grains online as well. Please check the appendix for a list of resources, including websites that sell active cultures like kefir grains. Once you have some, you can keep using them, saving them, and using them again for other batches.

Preparing kefir is quite simple. Place 1–2 tablespoons of kefir grains in a jar, crock, or container. Add 2 cups of milk. Then cover the container and let it ferment. After about 12 hours, you will see that the milk has thickened into kefir. Taste it, stopping the fermentation if it is ready or giving it a few more hours if needed. Before transferring it to the refrigerator, you must remove your kefir grains using a strainer. Have a second container ready to pour the kefir into, which you can use to store it in the fridge. Place the kefir grains back in your original container, add some more milk, and start the next batch. If you do not need a continuous culture, then you can store your kefir grains in the milk inside the refrigerator for up to two weeks before using them again.

There are dozens of recipes throughout this book that use yogurt and kefir. We'll just start off with a handful of savory soup and dip recipes here, which have cucumbers as their common thread.

Tzatziki Dip, Raita Sauce, and Chilled Kefir Soup

When you're eating a spicy meal, nothing cools like a cucumber. Combined with yogurt or kefir, cucumbers can make delicious raw sauces and soups. Creamy cucumber dishes can make refreshing accompaniments to spicy main courses. They can even make meals all by themselves. And you know they must be good, since the recipes here are drawn from four separate countries: Morocco, Greece, India, and Russia. For simplicity's sake, I have combined the Moroccan yogurt-cucumber dip and Indian raita with the Greek tzatziki, explaining their variations. The three are very similar dishes, differing only in which herbs and spices they use. There is a separate recipe for the kefir soup, though it features most of the same ingredients also.

Basic Recipe for Tzatziki Dip, Raita Sauce, and Moroccan Yogurt Sauce

Each recipe makes 2–3 cups

- 2 cups Greek yogurt (homemade yogurt strained in tight cheesecloth for 3–5 hours or in refrigerator overnight)
- 1 large English cucumber, split in half, seeded, and grated
- 1–2 cloves garlic, crushed
- 2 teaspoons sea salt
- Pinch of black pepper

Combine these basic ingredients with the additions of one of the three recipes below. Stir everything in well. Taste, adjust with more salt or spices as needed, and serve.

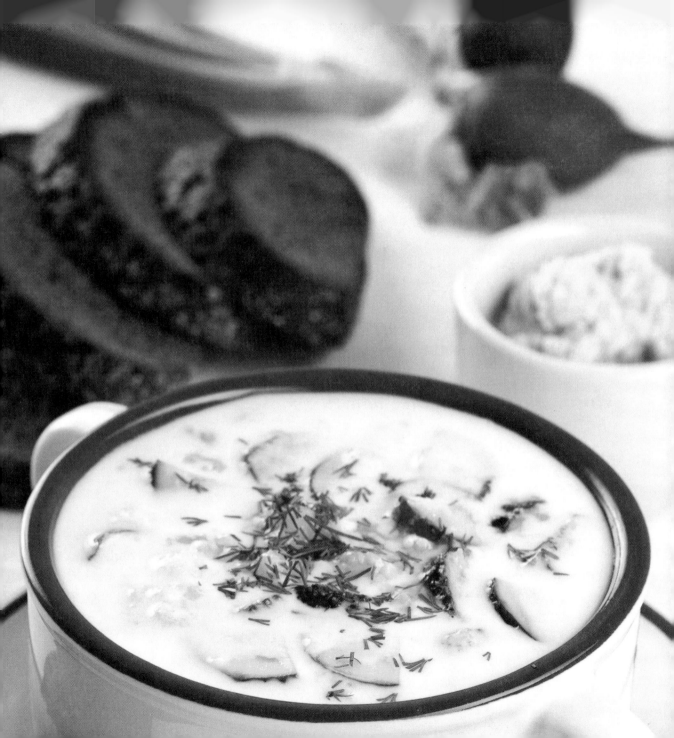

Tzatziki Dip additions

- 2–3 tablespoons lemon juice
- Zest of one lemon
- Optional: 1 tablespoon fresh dill, chopped

Raita Sauce additions

- ¼ cup cilantro, chopped
- ¼ cup scallions, chopped
- ½ teaspoon cumin or curry powder
- ¼ teaspoon cayenne of other chili pepper powder
- Optional: 1 large tomato, chopped

Moroccan Yogurt Sauce additions

- ¼ cup mint leaves, chopped
- ¼ cup parsley, chopped
- ½ teaspoon each: cumin, coriander powder
- ¼ teaspoon each: cinnamon, anise seed

Optional: If you have a Middle Eastern or North African grocery store nearby, see if it sells a spice blend called Ras El Hanout. This is a complex blend of up to thirty spices, including those in this recipe. Try using about 1 teaspoon of Ras El Hanout to replace the cumin, coriander powder, cinnamon, and anise seed in this recipe (as well as replace the black pepper in the basic recipe).

Kefir Soup (Russian Okroshka)

Makes about 4–6 cups

This recipe has been adapted from the *Cultures for Health* website, which is located at www.culturesforhealth.com and is an excellent source of fermentation supplies.

- 3–3½ cups kefir
- 1 large English cucumber, finely chopped or grated
- 1 bunch small radishes, cut in half and thinly sliced (or substitute 1–2 large carrots)
- ¼ cup chives, finely chopped (you can substitute scallions if you prefer)
- ¼ cup fresh dill, finely chopped
- 3 hard-boiled eggs, finely chopped
- 1 large beet, boiled or raw, grated
- Salt and pepper to taste
- Water, as needed to thin soup
- Optional: Substitute 1 medium potato (steamed or boiled) for beet
- Optional: Baby spinach (¼–½ cup), finely chopped

Combine 3 cups of kefir with other ingredients and stir. Add additional kefir or water as needed to thin soup to desired consistency. Season to taste with salt and pepper. Serve with warm rye bread.

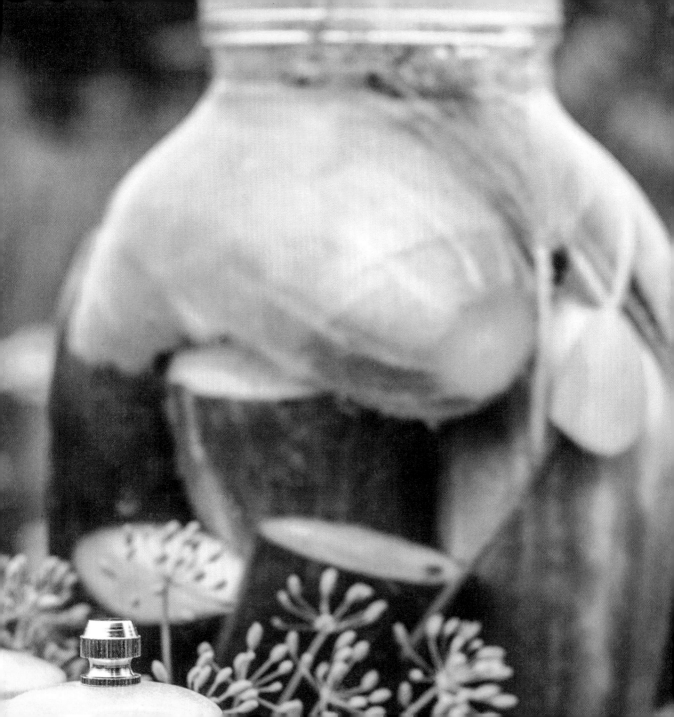

Chapter 6
Naturally Cultured Pickles

Have you ever tasted a naturally fermented dill pickle? It is crispier, crunchier, and has a fresher taste than any cucumber that has been embalmed with vinegar. Once you have tasted a natural pickle, it may be hard to go back to vinegar pickles. The one brand of commercial pickle that comes close to tasting natural is Clausen™; perhaps you have tried one and remarked that it is crispier than some others. This is because Clausen™ pickles begin their pickling journey in a naturally cultured brine before undergoing a secondary pickling stage in vinegar. The process keeps them crispier than most pickles, but unfortunately the culture is no longer active by the time you consume it, so these pickles are not probiotic.

Naturally cultured pickles are quite healthy for you, nourishing your body with beneficial bacteria and live food enzymes. Sadly, the pickles cured in vinegar are not always as healthy. Besides being harder to digest, many commercial brands of pickles contain chemical preservatives and artificial coloring. The most common dye used in pickles, FD&C Yellow #5, has been linked with more allergic reactions than any other coloring agent.

Just stick to natural pickles. They have plenty of flavor and a much more beautiful color. You do not need any of these unnatural additives. You also may find that your family is healthier after you cut out some of the chemically preserved foods from your diet.

The process of natural pickling goes back several thousand years. The recipe may have come from the Indus River civilization in India, along with cucumber seeds.

Around 2000 BC, people in Mesopotamia were making pickles, which the ancient Egyptians also enjoyed. Cucumbers were mentioned twice in the Bible. Aristotle and Cleopatra raved about the health benefits associated with eating pickles. Generals from Julius Caesar to Napoleon believed pickles were healthy for their troops. Queen Elizabeth enjoyed them as well. Shakespeare made puns about pickles in several of his plays. George Washington had a collection of 476 different kinds of cucumbers. And Thomas Jefferson wrote that there was "nothing more comforting than a finely spiced pickle . . . from the aromatic jar below the stairs of Aunt Sally's cellar."

The process for making naturally cultured pickles is very simple. Basically, you wash, trim, and cut (to your preferred size) some fresh pickling cucumbers. You can use other vegetables as well, including carrots, radishes, and zucchini squash, but cucumbers are most people's favorites. Put these in a jar, fill it nearly to the top with water, and then add plenty of sea salt. Making your own pickles gives you a great opportunity to flavor them however you want. The basic flavoring ingredients generally include dill, peppercorns, mustard, and garlic, but you are welcome to increase or decrease the quantities of these, which is suggested in the recipes. And of course you can add other herbs and spices that you like.

Natural Dill Pickles

Makes a 1-quart jar of pickles

This is the classic dill pickle recipe. Feel free to tinker with it, adjusting the herbs and seasonings as you wish. For example, you may want to add some extra garlic or spice. You will need a one-quart jar or fermenting crock.

- 2½ cups water
- 1 pound pickling cucumbers (whole, sliced, or cut lengthwise into four spears each)
- 1–2 heads or sprigs of fresh dill (in a pinch, you can substitute 1/3 cup to ½ cup dried dill, but quality will vary)
- 3 cloves garlic, crushed or finely chopped
- ¼ cup onion, sliced or chopped
- 2 grape leaves
- 1 bay leaf
- 1½ tablespoons sea salt
- ¼ teaspoon coriander seeds
- ¼ teaspoon peppercorns
- ¼ teaspoon mustard seeds
- Optional: 1 small red chili pepper (whole or sliced in half), ¼ teaspoon turmeric powder (to add yellow color and antioxidants)

You probably will need a little less than one pound of cucumbers, but the actual quantity will depend on how you cut them and pack them in the jar. Wash cukes well and cut off the tips from both ends. Then cut or slice them if desired (sliced or quartered/speared cucumbers will ferment more quickly). Dissolve the sea salt in the water. Add the garlic, onions, salt, and all herbs and spices to the bottom of the crock or jar. Then pack it with cucumbers. Cover with salt brine water, making sure to completely cover the cucumbers but still leaving a little space on top of the container. Cover and let pickles ferment. If any scum forms on top of the brine water during fermentation, just scrape it off. After 3 days, check them and make sure that you can see bubbles rising. If you like really fresh pickles, you can taste them in 3–4 days. If you prefer them sour, it may take as long as 10 days, but probably less. Just taste and move them to the refrigerator as soon as the taste is right for you. They will last for weeks in the fridge.

Dilly Beans and Carrot Sticks

Makes a 1-quart jar of pickled vegetables

Dilly Beans are a popular homemade pickled dish, which you can make with a cultured fermentation. If you've had enough of dill, you can substitute any other fresh herbs that you like (or just leave this out). This recipe incorporates some carrot sticks also, but you can use 100 percent green beans if you prefer. You will need a one-quart jar or fermenting crock.

- 3 quarts water for blanching + 1 quart for brine
- 1 pound fresh green beans (snap beans)
- 2 large carrots, cut into long sticks about the same size as the beans
- 3 garlic cloves, crushed
- 1 tablespoon fresh dill, chopped, or 1 teaspoon dried dill
- 1 teaspoon mustard seeds
- 1 small chili pepper, sliced (or whole, if dried)
- 1 grape leaf
- 1 tablespoon sea salt + more to taste

Blanching Vegetables
(Optional; improves flavor and appearance)

In a large pan, bring 3 quarts of water to a boil. Put green beans in the boiling water for 1 minute, add carrot sticks, and give them 1 more minute (2 minutes total for beans). Then strain vegetables out immediately and cool them. You can do this by transferring them to an ice-water bath or rinsing them under cold water in the sink.

Making Pickles

Place cooled beans and carrots in a jar or other container, add garlic, salt, herbs, and water. Cover, shake, and let the vegetables ferment at room temperature for about 3–4 days, checking them periodically. Feel free to taste them and move to the refrigerator when you think they are ready to eat. The Dilly Beans and Carrot Sticks last for at least two months in the fridge, during which time they will continue to ferment and sour slowly.

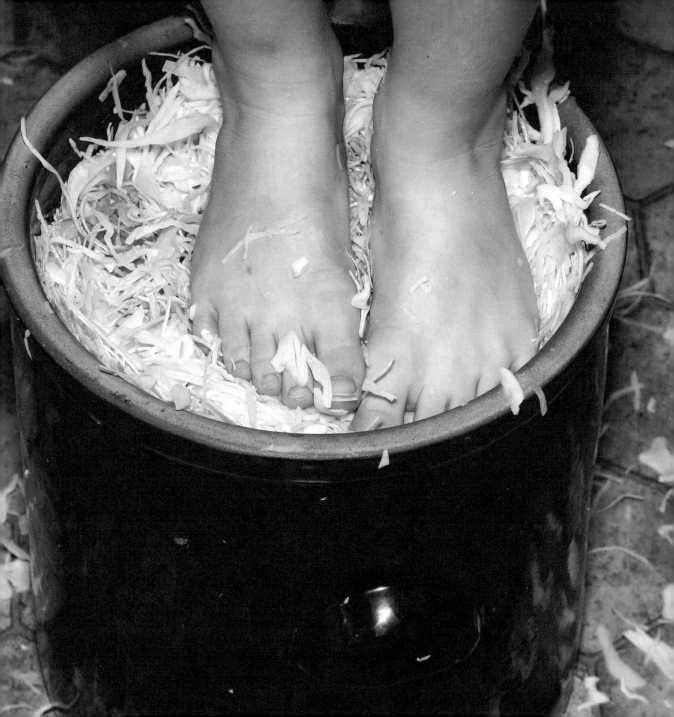

Chapter 7
Sauerkraut

Ah, kraut time. You knew it was in this book, right? You could smell it fermenting a mile away. Like kimchi and other naturally fermented vegetable dishes, sauerkraut can be pungent. In temperate climates throughout the world, beneficial lactobacteria seem to agree on one thing: cabbage is great stuff. If you feed them cabbage, they will turn it deliciously pungent.

What's good for them is good for us. Sauerkraut contains fresh vegetables as well as live probiotics, nourishing our whole bodies with vitamins, minerals, enzymes, and antioxidants while building the health of our digestive systems. It's no wonder so many people swear that sauerkraut has cured them of some imbalance or disease. Candida, cancer, vaginal yeast infections, diabetes, diverticulitis, eczema, and arthritis are a few ailments that many people claim can be treated effectively by consuming sauerkraut.

I will not go as far as to recommend sauerkraut as a treatment; you can discuss this with a qualified physician or natural health practitioner. But it seems pretty likely that restoring a healthy balance in your digestive system might directly help correct imbalances like indigestion, candida, and yeast infections. At the same time, a major influx of vitamins, minerals, enzymes, antioxidants, and probiotics should have a positive effect on your body's health. If your body is stronger, hopefully your immune system can stave off most diseases on its own.

Just as yogurt and kefir may have had the same ancestor, sauerkraut and kimchi probably did as well. The process of pickling cabbage to preserve it apparently started in China or Central Asia. Initially, the cabbage was pickled in wine to preserve it before someone had the bright idea to try pickling it in salt brine. This allowed naturally present lactobacteria to flourish and create the fermentation.

Genghis Khan and his troops were known to use pickled cabbage, and they may even have been the ones who started using salt water instead of wine. Early on, it became clear that preserving vegetables helped store their nutrition, which could be taken on the road by the nomadic Mongols and their soldiers. If the Mongols were the first to use lactofermentation for sauerkraut/kimchi, they probably also discovered that the natural fermentation helped them digest meat, which made up much of their diet. However, lactofermented vegetables have been used in one form or another for many thousands of years in Europe, so it is possible that someone in Europe began to ferment sauerkraut without the use of wine.

Did you know that Hungarian and Korean are related languages? Look at a map and try to figure that one out. In fact, this language group has the same common thread as the sauerkraut of Central/Eastern Europe and the kimchi of Korea: the Mongols. Like their language, they spread their fermented foods across the Eurasian continent. Fermented cabbage developed a following on both ends of this huge landmass, eventually turning into European sauerkraut and Asian kimchi.

Basic sauerkraut consists of shredded cabbage, salt, and perhaps a little extra water. That's it. You put the shredded cabbage in a jar, clay pot, or crock, add salt, and wait until this draws out the natural juices of the cabbage. This liquid should be enough to submerge the cabbage completely, but if not, you can add a little more water and salt. Then you let this sit while the lactobacteria do their work.

Speaking of lactobacteria, do you need to add any culture? Most kraut makers do not add any special culture, relying instead on naturally present bacteria to ferment the cabbage. If you prefer the greater speed and certainty of a culture, you can add your own. There are two simple sources for kefir culture. The first is kefir grains (or a few tablespoons of water kefir, even without the grains). The second is yogurt whey (liquid) from some good quality sour yogurt that contains active cultures. Both of these cultures make very effective sauerkraut starters and will speed up the natural fermentation by a day or two.

Sauerkraut fermentation usually takes about 4–10 days. The actual length of time can depend on the air temperature (it moves faster in warmer weather), the strength of the culture, and how sour you like it. You are welcome to steal a taste of your kraut every day or so with a clean spoon. Once the sauerkraut is ripe enough for your tastes, go ahead and refrigerate it. Refrigeration slows down the fermentation process to a crawl, so it will continue to ripen over time. Kept in a sealed container, such as a jar, kraut will last for months in the refrigerator while you eat it.

If, at any point, you see a mold-like white film on the surface of the sauerkraut, just wipe it off with a paper towel or skim off the top layer and throw it away. It probably is not mold but a yeast bloom, which is totally natural. The rest of your kraut should be just fine.

Today, sauerkraut remains a major food item in Germany, the Netherlands, Poland, and other countries in Central and Eastern Europe. In many of these locations, sauerkraut typically is eaten with meat, such as sausages and pork. From Russia to the border provinces of Alsace-Lorraine in France to Pennsylvania's Dutch country, sauerkraut remains a beloved food. As modern evidence mounts that naturally fermented foods are healthy, there has been a renewed interest in sauerkraut. Today, people are rediscovering this food that their parents or grandparents fed them as kids, while members of younger generations are tasting sauerkraut for the first time.

Sauerkraut

Makes 3–4 cups

Begin with a head of cabbage, either the light green or the purple kind. In addition to a crock or jar for fermenting, you will need something with which to weigh down the cabbage. If you are using a jar (which usually has a narrower opening than a crock), then you can use a mixing bowl (preferably nonmetallic) for the first part and weigh down the cabbage with a smaller bowl that has something heavy inside of it. If you are using a crock, then use something that fits inside of it as a weight. Basically, you just need to make sure the shredded cabbage stays under the water level for the first 24 hours, and after that the kraut can handle itself.

- 1 head of cabbage
- 1–2 tablespoons sea salt
- Water, if needed
- Optional: grated or thinly sliced carrots, caraway seeds
- 2 tablespoons liquid culture, such as yogurt whey, sauerkraut or natural pickle juice, or water kefir

Wash the head of cabbage and shred it. You can shred cabbage just by slicing it thinly on a cutting board. Otherwise, you can use a food processor or mandolin grater.

Place the shredded cabbage in the mixing bowl. Cover the cabbage with 1–2 tablespoons of salt, plus the culture ingredient (if you wish to use one), and use your clean hands to mix these in very well.

Using your hands, push down the cabbage shreds in the bowl or crock. Try to squeeze out a bit of the liquid from the leaves, which the salt will draw out.

Use your weight to weigh down the cabbage as much as possible to continue squeezing out the fluid. In the first 24 hours, put your washed hands in three to four times to squeeze down the cabbage. The fluid should reach the top of the cabbage after a while, but if it doesn't, you can add a little nonchlorinated water and another pinch or two of sea salt.

After 24 hours, if you have used a bowl, then you can move the cabbage to your jar. Make sure to pour the fluid from the bowl over it also. Whether you use a jar or crock, the cabbage shreds should all be sitting at or under the fluid level now. Any cabbage sticking above the fluid will invite mold.

Put your kraut in a quiet place, cover it loosely, and let it ferment. Check it every day. After 3 days, your kraut may be ready. Taste and see if you like it this fresh. If not, let it go a little longer. Four to ten days is a typical time window, after which you can move the sauerkraut to your refrigerator, where it will last for months.

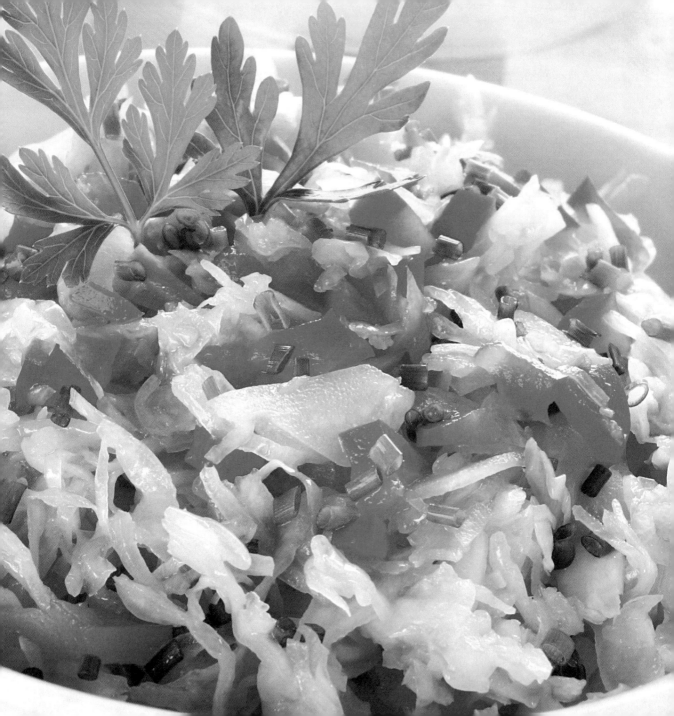

Salvadoran Curtido (Central American Sauerkraut)

Makes 5–6 cups

This Latin American fermented dish is a nice spicy alternative to the plainer sour-salty taste of regular sauerkraut. Basically, it is a sauerkraut recipe with the additions of garlic, onions, jalapeno peppers, and herbs such as oregano or cilantro. For a milder version, replace the jalapenos with sweet bell pepper instead. Nowadays, many people make this dish with vinegar, but as with sauerkraut, pickles, and many other dishes, natural lactofermentation is the healthier method.

- 2 heads cabbage, shredded
- 2 large carrots, grated or shredded
- 2 cloves garlic, crushed
- 1 large onion, thinly sliced, or 4–6 scallions, chopped
- 2–3 tablespoons jalapeno peppers (2–3 medium peppers), diced (spicy version), or ¼ cup red bell pepper, chopped (mild version)
- 1 teaspoon dried oregano, or 1 bunch fresh cilantro, chopped
- 3–4 tablespoons sea salt
- 2 tablespoons liquid culture, such as yogurt whey, sauerkraut or natural pickle juice, or water kefir
- Optional: ½ cup fresh pineapple, chopped

In a large bowl or crock, mix together shredded cabbage with the other ingredients. Then follow directions for making sauerkraut, above.

Sauerkraut Wrap

Makes 1 wrap sandwich

Here is one easy way to use sauerkraut in a healthy wrap sandwich.

- 1 large whole-grain tortilla
- 1 handful of lettuce, baby leaves or chopped
- 1–3 tablespoons sauerkraut
- ¼–½ cup hummus or meat of your choice
- ¼ cup chopped tomatoes or sliced cucumbers
- Spread/sauce of your choice: mayonnaise, mustard, pasta sauce, salsa, ketchup, salad dressing, etc.
- Optional: cheese, sliced avocado, sliced mushrooms, sprouts, sliced olives or pickles, chopped parsley, cilantro, or mint

Place all ingredients in a line down the middle of your tortilla. Wrap up sides into a burrito shape and enjoy.

Broccoli Krautslaw

Makes 3–4 cups of slaw

- 2 heads of broccoli
- 2 large carrots
- ½ bell pepper
- ¼ cup chives (or ½ red onion or ¼ cup scallions), finely chopped

- 1 cup sauerkraut, or curtido
- Your favorite salad dressing, to taste (see the separate salad dressing recipes in this book)
- Optional: ¼ cup natural pickles or olives, finely chopped
- Optional: raisins, chopped walnuts, almonds, or other nuts

Chop or grate all ingredients by hand or using a food processor. Toss in a covered container with your favorite dressing. Let this ferment/marinate at room temperature for a few hours, then transfer it to the refrigerator. It will be delicious right away, but even better the next day.

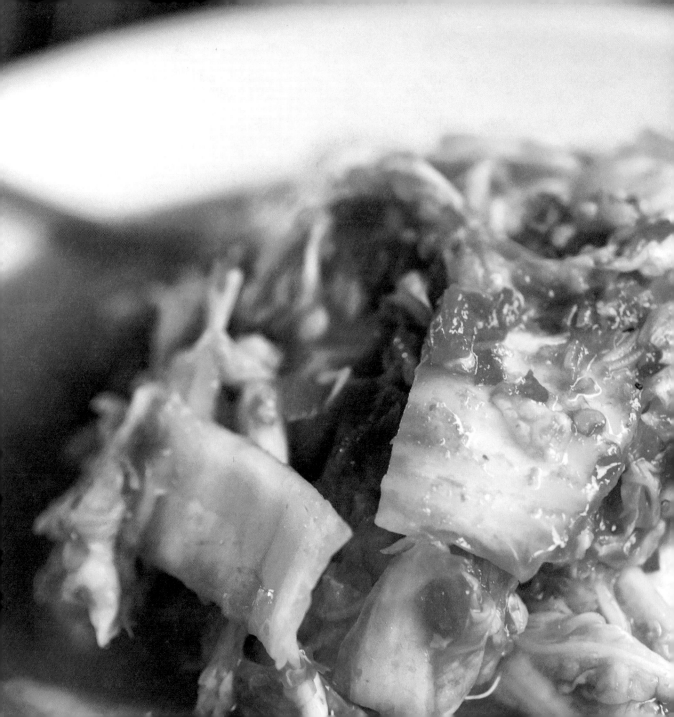

Chapter 8
Kimchi

Kimchi is one of the crown jewels of fermented foods. The popularity of this spicy, pickled side dish has grown worldwide in recent years. But the Koreans themselves have known for many years about the amazing health benefits of their national dish.

The practice of lactofermenting vegetables must have spread east with the Mongols just as it spread west to Europe. Fermented vegetables took firm root in Korea, a peninsula that enjoys nearly subtropical summers but also fiercely frozen winters. During this time of year, native sources of fresh food were scarce, and kimchi filled an important need.

Kimchi is prepared rather like sauerkraut, except with the additions of crushed garlic, ground chili peppers, and other seasonings like green onions and ginger. The most common base ingredient is Napa cabbage, sometimes known as Chinese cabbage. Cucumber and Daikon radish kimchis are also prevalent, along with less common side dishes like burdock root kimchi or perilla leaf kimchi. Less common supporting ingredients can include pine nuts, slices of Asian pear, sour green plums, or oysters. Ingredients can be added chopped or whole. Fermented shrimp or anchovy paste usually serves as the starter culture, generally including the unique species of lactobacteria known as *L. kimchii*, though a slower fermentation can occur by just letting the naturally present lactobacteria do their job. All in all, there are more than one hundred kinds of kimchi, including cold soups made in water brine called "water kimchi."

Kimchi is dear to the heart of Korea's national consciousness. The average Korean consumes forty pounds (more than eighteen kilograms) of it per year. Anyone you meet in Korea, where I lived for more than two years, swears by kimchi's health benefits. Visitors may question some of the claims, since it seems like kimchi becomes a subject in almost every conversation, but its effects on improved digestion and immunity have been supported by several studies. It also packs a huge density of vitamins A and C, B complex vitamins, minerals, antioxidants, and enzymes into every bite. Kimchi is a superfood and they are right to be proud of it.

Not only do Koreans enjoy kimchi as a raw side dish but they also use it to flavor many cooked dishes, including stews, noodles, dumplings, and fried rice. I have included two of these recipes, both of which are not cooked after the kimchi has been added. Most families still make their own kimchi at least once a year, many of them using the huge, traditional clay pots known as kimchi pots. When prepared in the warm days of early autumn, kimchi can be stored in these pots in the cold winter weather, though some kinds of kimchi are made at other times of the year.

Napa Cabbage Kimchi

As with sauerkraut, you will need a large jar or fermenting crock to make kimchi. This recipe will require two (preferably large) mixing bowls, one large and the other smaller.

- 1 large Napa cabbage, preferably organic
- 2 tablespoons sea salt
- 2–3 green onions or scallions

- 1 clove garlic, minced or crushed
- ⅔ cup hot red pepper powder
- ½ tablespoon sugar
- 2 tablespoons liquid culture, such as yogurt whey, sauerkraut or natural pickle juice, or water kefir

Take the outer layer of leaves off the Napa cabbage and discard. Wash the remaining cabbage well.

Chop the leaves. Their size should be similar to chopped lettuce in a typical salad.

Place the chopped cabbage in the large bowl. Sprinkle in a little sea salt, rub it into the leaves, and mix together.

In the smaller bowl, mix the crushed garlic, red pepper powder, sugar, remaining salt, and optional culture. This should form a pasty sauce. Add a spoonful or two of nonchlorinated water if it seems too dry.

Pour the sauce paste over the chopped cabbage. Add the chopped green onion. Toss gently until it is coated.

Put the kimchi mixture in a glass jar or crock. Cover it loosely with the lid or a cloth. Once the kimchi begins to give off a fermenting smell, probably in 2–3 days, then taste it. As soon as you believe it is ready, you can cover the container and move it to the refrigerator. The fermentation generally takes 3–10 days. Your kimchi will continue to ferment slowly in the refrigerator, where it will last for weeks or months (depending on how sour you can handle it!).

Radish Kimchi (Korean Kkaktugi)

While cabbage kimchi is the most well-known, there are other types also. One particular favorite is Radish kimchi. This recipe utilizes fermented shrimp paste as a source of lactobacteria, though you can substitute less authentic sources such as yogurt whey, sauerkraut juice, or vegetable culture. Both the shrimp paste and fish stock are available at Asian grocery stores. The sea salt in this recipe is used to coat and leech fluid from the radish cubes, but it is then rinsed off, so there is no added salt in the end product. If you decide to make this side dish without fermented shrimp paste, which is salty, then you may need to add additional sea salt near the end (to suit your taste).

- 2 large Korean Daikon radishes (larger than most other types), cut into 1-inch cubes
- 1 large onion, sliced or roughly chopped
- 5–7 scallions (green onions), finely chopped
- 5–7 cloves garlic
- 2 inches ginger, peeled and finely chopped
- ⅓ cup dried red chili pepper powder
- ⅓ cup fermented shrimp paste
- ⅓ cup fish stock or fish sauce (such as anchovy)
- 4–5 tablespoons sea salt
- 1½ tablespoons sugar
- More salt, to taste
- Sesame seeds, to sprinkle on top

Trim Daikon radishes and cut them into cubes. Place radish cubes in a bowl, add salt, and mix well. Let them sit for 1 hour, during which time the salt will leech out some of the fluid. After 1 hour, rinse radishes and drain them in a colander or

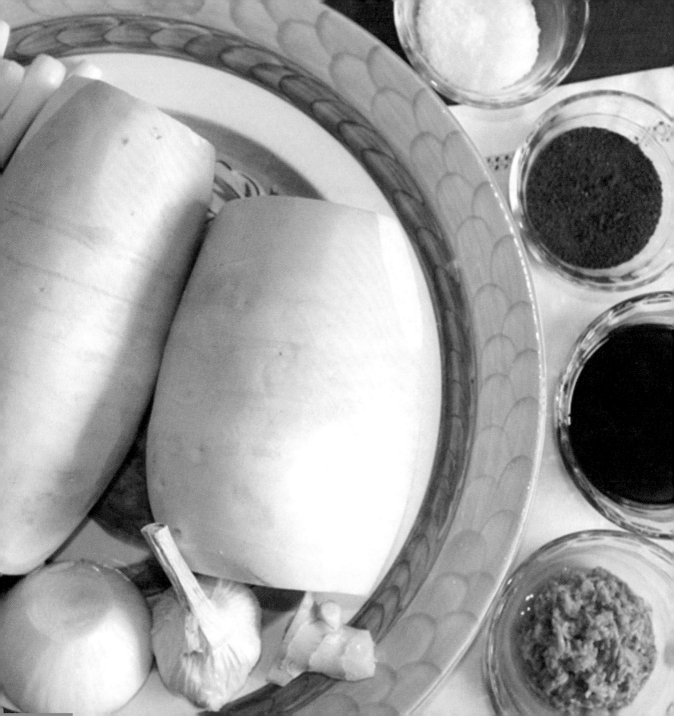

strainer. Use a blender to combine and purée the onion, garlic, ginger, and shrimp paste with the fish stock to make a thin paste. In a bowl, mix onion-garlic-ginger purée with fermented shrimp paste, fish stock, sugar, and chili pepper powder. Toss this sauce mixture with the radish cubes, coating them evenly. Then stir in scallions. Move radish kimchi to a large crock or jar, pouring and scraping over it any additional sauce that remains in the bowl. Cover and let kimchi ferment at room temperature. It should take 2–4 days, depending on temperature, but check it every day or so and feel free to taste. Once it has fermented, cover tightly and move to the refrigerator for storage. You can keep eating it and the kimchi will last for several weeks in the fridge.

Kimchi Bibimbap (Mixed Vegetable Rice)

Makes 1–2 servings

This is the probiotic version of the traditional Korean mixed rice meal known as bibimbap (pronounced "bee-bim-bop"). Essentially, cooked rice is served with a variety of stir-fried and raw vegetables, mushrooms, and bean sprouts, as well as a fried egg and/or ground beef. The person eating it simply adds in as much Korean hot sauce (gochujang) as he or she wants, then mixes up the whole dish in a big bowl and eats it. Koreans eat kimchi on the side, but our recipe adds this into the dish directly. This means that you get to decide whether you need any additional hot sauce (which you can do after mixing and tasting it). If it is spicy enough for you already, then adding a little extra soy sauce and/or sesame oil will give you enough moisture and flavor.

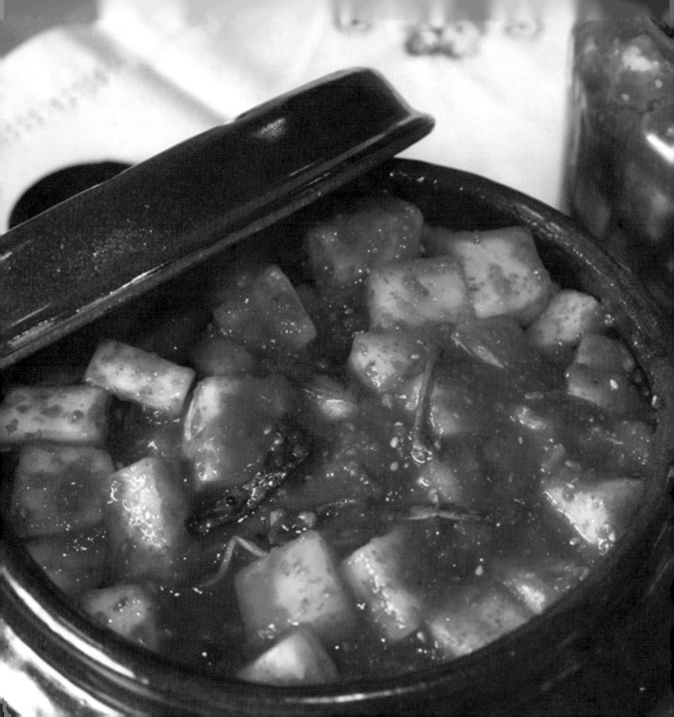

You can find all ingredients at an Asian grocery store. If you cannot find all of the vegetables/sprouts/mushrooms, etc., then just use what you have. Once you have at least three of these ingredients plus kimchi, go ahead and give this dish a try.

Start by cooking some rice (as a whole food person, I recommend brown rice, but you could use white rice, preferably the sticky sushi kind). For 100 percent raw food diets, soak and sprout some brown rice or wild rice to get it tender enough for eating. Personally, I am not able to eat large quantities of raw grains and I am not convinced that even soaked and sprouted rice is safe to eat in large amounts, but I will leave this up to you. Wild rice is fairly tender (like a wheatberry) once it has been properly soaked and sprouted, so if that alternative appeals to you, please seek more information online about preparing wild rice for raw food diets.

- 1½ cups cooked rice
- ½ cup bean sprouts (soybean and/or mung bean)
- ½ cup kimchi, chopped (more, to taste)
- ½ cup carrot, grated or cut into long, very thin strips
- ½ cup spinach, sautéed with a little garlic
- 5 shiitake mushrooms, chopped and sautéed with a little garlic
- 1 teaspoon sesame oil (the toasted variety has the best flavor)
- Korean hot sauce (gochujang) or soy sauce, to taste
- Optional: 1 fried egg, ½ cup ground beef (cooked), ½ teaspoon sesame seeds

Part of the joy of eating bibimbap is getting to mix it yourself after seeing all the ingredients displayed separately in the bowl. Use a large bowl that someone can eat from. You will fill it nearly to the top, but leave enough space to allow the ingredients to be stirred. Put the cooked rice in the bowl first. Cover the rice with the fried egg, if you use one. Place the other ingredients on top of this, each in its own separate section or corner (not overlapping much). Over the top, sprinkle in the ground beef or sesame seeds (both optional) and drizzle a little sesame oil. Before eating, add some hot sauce or soy sauce, then break up the egg and mix up your dish as well as you can with a spoon. Yum!

Kimchi Noodles

Makes 1–2 servings

This recipe begins with your favorite noodles. Wheat noodles, either Asian or Western types, work best. Spaghetti, fettuccini, macaroni, or any raw food substitute should be fine.

- 2 cups cooked noodles
- ½–1 cup kimchi, chopped
- 1 teaspoon toasted sesame oil
- 1 teaspoon sesame seeds
- ½ cucumber, sliced lengthwise into thin ribbons that resemble noodles
- Soy sauce or salt to taste
- Optional: 1 sheet of sushi seaweed

Put fresh cooked noodles in a bowl, add other ingredients, and stir. This actually is a great cold dish, but if you need to warm them up, then stir-fry the noodles first in a little cooking oil on a skillet. While they are still warm, but no longer scalding hot, transfer to a bowl, then add other ingredients and stir. If you use the optional sheet of sushi seaweed, then crumble this over the top of your dish at the last minute just before eating.

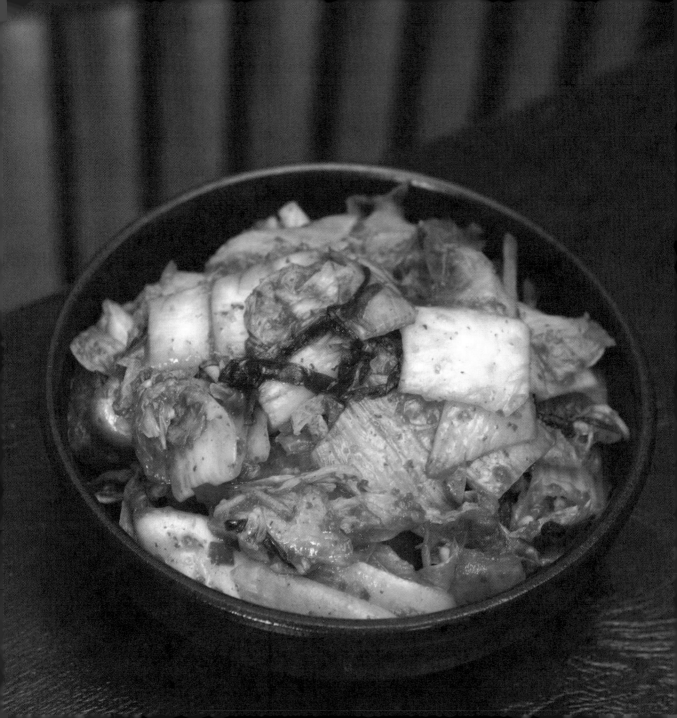

Chapter 9
Other Fermented Vegetable, Fruit, Grain, Carb, and Protein Dishes

You are not limited to cabbage and cucumbers. There are dozens of other vegetables, not to mention fruits, grains, and other foods, that can be fermented with a probiotic culture. In general, firmer vegetables and fruits hold up better than soft ones in fermentation. Carrots, beets, celery, onions, fennel, garlic, green beans, radishes, jicama, and cauliflower are examples of relatively firm vegetables, while apples, cranberries, peaches, and plums are some good fruits to try in chutneys, relishes, and jams.

Grains and other carbohydrates can ferment well also. After all, breads and beers are fermented with yeast, and both are grain-based. However, probiotic grain dishes are rarer than fermented dairy and vegetable dishes. Fermented porridges are staples in Africa and we have one recipe here for a porridge drink. Rejuvelac is another grain-fermented drink that is an American health beverage. Poi, the traditional Hawaiian and Polynesian dish, involves fermenting the starchy taro root. There is a fermented Corn Salsa recipe here as well.

Fermenting proteins, such as beans, eggs, and meats, is more difficult because the species of organisms we consider probiotic are not necessarily the same ones needed to ferment proteins. Italian salami and Chinese thousand-year-old eggs are some examples of fermented proteins, but the process tends to be complex and not necessarily probiotic. I have included a handful of simple-to-prepare probiotic protein dishes, some of which simply involve adding yogurt, sauerkraut, or another source of probiotics to your food before consuming it.

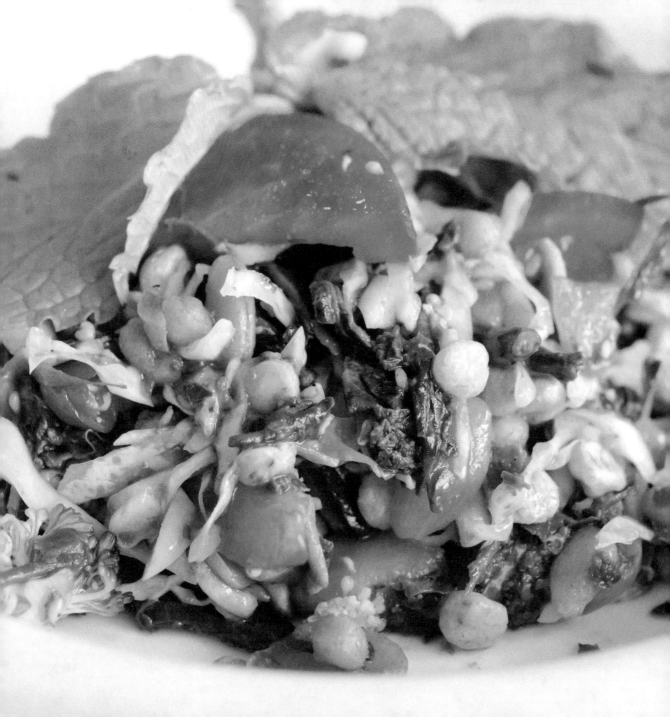

Fermented Green Tea Salad (Burmese Lahpet)

Makes 1 family-sized "salad"

If you like drinking green tea, have you ever thought of eating it? If you can find a Burmese restaurant, this traditional dish usually appears on the menu. Though it is considered a salad, this dish is quite heavy and high in protein. Enjoy lahpet with rice, as a side dish, or mixed with additional cabbage or lettuce to make a healthy, nutty salad. I have adapted the basic recipe somewhat to make it a bit lighter (the original version is very high in fat and calories due to all the nuts, seeds, and deep-fried beans). I also have substituted sauerkraut for the cabbage, but you can use plain, unfermented cabbage if you prefer. This is a great way to use leftover tea leaves if you make your own whole leaf green tea. If you are not a green tea drinker, then you can steam some green tea leaves for 5–10 minutes or soak them in hot water for 2–3 hours. Note that the measurement for green tea leaves refers to the proper quantity of *dried* tea leaves; these will expand a good deal once soaked or steamed.

Fermented tea leaves:

- ½ cup dry green tea leaves (use a whole-leaf tea), steamed or soaked
- ½ inch ginger, peeled and finely minced
- 2–3 cloves garlic, crushed
- 2 tablespoons yogurt whey, water kefir, or vegetable culture
- ½ teaspoon salt

Additional salad ingredients:

- ½ cup sauerkraut
- 3 large red tomatoes, cut into 1–2-inch pieces
- ¼ cup broccoli, raw or blanched, cut into 1–2-inch pieces
- 2 tablespoons roasted peanuts
- 2 tablespoons roasted pumpkin seeds
- 2 tablespoons roasted sesame seeds
- ¼ cup cooked garbanzo beans (chickpeas)
- ¼ cup cooked beans (preferably lima or butter beans, but you can use pinto, black, or kidney)

Optional: Traditional Lahpet uses dried shrimp, which I have replaced with broccoli. Also, feel free to increase the quantities of the nuts and seeds, which I have cut down by about 50 percent each due to the high caloric content of the final product. To make this spicy, you can add chopped green chilies or dried red pepper flakes.

Dressing:

You may not need much dressing if you use sauerkraut. Mix approximately equal parts lime juice, soy sauce, and either peanut oil or sesame oil, going lighter on the soy sauce if you have used sauerkraut and/or if any of your nuts or seeds are presalted. You can vary these proportions to taste, including a little honey or sugar in your dressing if you prefer a sweeter version.

After cooling the soaked or steamed green tea leaves, place them on a cutting board and cut each leaf in half. Place in a container or bowl, add crushed garlic, ginger, salt, lemon juice, and culture, mix this up, and cover the container or bowl. Let it ferment at room temperature for 24–48 hours.

In a salad bowl, mix together fermented tea leaves with other ingredients. Taste before adding any dressing, and then add as much as you need. Lahpet will keep in the refrigerator for at least a week, so you don't need to eat it all at once!

Marinated Mushrooms

Makes about 2½ cups

If you love marinated mushrooms, try out this fermented favorite. The mushrooms are cooked in this recipe, but if you prefer to leave them raw, just skip the cooking step and combine all ingredients in a jar or container (leaving out the onion if you wish). I cook them because mushrooms have a lot of air in them and I worry that leaving any air pockets could result in contamination. Cooking also yields a more uniform, marinated texture. This recipe uses a water sauté for the cooking, after which you can dump both the mushrooms and the cooked fluid into the ferment.

- 1 pound mushrooms, washed and halved or quartered
- ½ cup onion, chopped
- ½ cup water for cooking
- Small handful of fresh herbs of your choice, such as thyme, marjoram, oregano, dill, or rosemary
- 3 cups water
- 2 cloves garlic, crushed
- 1 tablespoon salt
- 2 teaspoons whey or starter culture

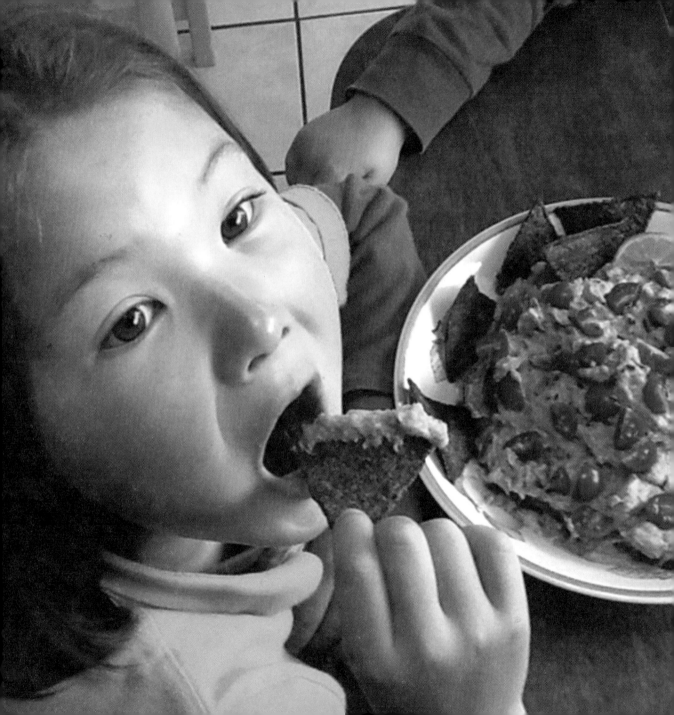

First, sauté mushrooms and onions in water until onions are translucent and mushrooms are soft. After cooling these to room temperature, move the mushrooms and cooking fluid into a jar or container. Dissolve the salt in the remaining water. Add all other ingredients and then fill (to one inch below the top) with the salt water. Cover loosely and let the 'shrooms ferment at room temperature for 3 days. Then cover and refrigerate for up to one or two weeks.

Sauer Guacamole Dip

Makes 4–6 servings

3–4 ripe avocadoes

- ½ cup sauerkraut, finely chopped
- Juice of ½ lemon or lime (start with less and increase it to taste)
- ½ teaspoon garlic powder
- 1 teaspoon chives or scallion, finely chopped
- ¼ cup tomato or red bell pepper, diced
- 2 tablespoons yogurt
- Sea salt, to taste
- Optional: handful of fresh cilantro, finely chopped

Peel avocadoes and mash them with a fork, adding lemon juice right away to prevent them from turning brown (oxidizing). Stir in other ingredients. Taste and adjust salt to your liking. If you eat this with salted tortilla chips, remember that your dip may not need much salt.

Corn Salsa

Makes about 4 cups

Probiotic corn salsa provides a taste of Latin America with a cultured twist. Fresh summer corn makes a great addition to salsa. If you would like, you can add cooked black beans to this dish for a true Southwest dip. For a mild version that is more like a relish, omit the chopped jalapeno peppers and cayenne pepper powder. If you use probiotic pickle juice as a starter culture, then you will need less salt than if your starter culture is yogurt whey or water kefir.

As with some other recipes, the probiotic part comes from adding yogurt or kefir culture when you make the salsa. But you are welcome to let it marinate and ferment for a longer period of time if you wish. This turns the corn slightly sour and increases the probiotic content. If you opt for a longer ferment, then I recommend holding the chopped tomatoes and cilantro, adding these after the fermentation is complete, since they do not hold up as well as the corn.

- 1½ cups fresh corn (cut from the cob)
- 1½ cups fresh tomatoes, chopped
- ¼ cup red onions or scallions, diced
- ½ cup cilantro, chopped
- ¼ cup peppers, chopped
- Jalapeno pepper, diced (to taste, 1 teaspoon to 1 tablespoon)
- 1 clove garlic, crushed or diced

- Sea salt, pepper, cayenne pepper to taste
- Juice of 1 lime
- 2–3 tablespoons starter culture
- 1 tablespoon olive oil
- Optional: ¼ cup cooked black beans

Place all ingredients (except tomatoes, cilantro, and olive oil) into a bowl or container, and stir with a spoon, making sure to coat all the corn and vegetables with the probiotic starter culture fluid. Add ½ teaspoon salt, taste it, and then add more salt if needed. This will not be the final salting opportunity, but you want a tasty brine for the fermentation. Also add as much chopped jalapeno and chili pepper powder as you wish. Then cover the bowl or container, put it in a quiet place, and let it sit for 6–12 hours.

Uncover the bowl or container. Check to see how much fluid is at the bottom. If there is an inch or more of fluid, pour some out or ladle it out with a spoon (you can discard or use this as starter for something else). You want this dish to be somewhat wet, but not swimming in brine! Then stir in the tomato, cilantro, and olive oil, taste it again, and adjust the final saltiness and spiciness to taste. Enjoy with chips.

Dolmas (Grape Leaves Stuffed with Herbed Rice)

Makes about 16–24 dolmas (depending on size of leaf wraps)

Dolmas are a traditional food of the Mediterranean region, particularly popular in Greece and Turkey. There are many variations, some using ground lamb and others using dried currants or raisins. Most dolmas have a sour-salty flavor accented by dill, mint, cumin, allspice, and/or other flavors. Traditionally, lemon juice or vinegar is used to achieve the sour taste, but this recipe uses lactofermentation as well.

This is a two-step recipe. Step one involves fermenting the grape leaves, which serve as the wraps for the rice dish. Since there are various types of grapes that grow from the tropics to the far north, hopefully you can pick these fresh. For step one, I have borrowed from the fermented grape leaves recipe in Sally Fallon Morell's excellent book, *Nourishing Traditions.* Step two, the rice recipe, is mine. It uses some yogurt, so you do not need to ferment the whole dish separately unless you wish to do so. As always, you are free to take this in another direction by making it sweeter (add dried currants or raisins), saltier (add kalamata olives), or nuttier (add chopped almonds or pine nuts).

Step one: Fermented Grape Leaves

- 24 grape leaves, medium sized
- 1 tablespoon sea salt
- 4 tablespoons whey/cultured liquid
- 2 cups water

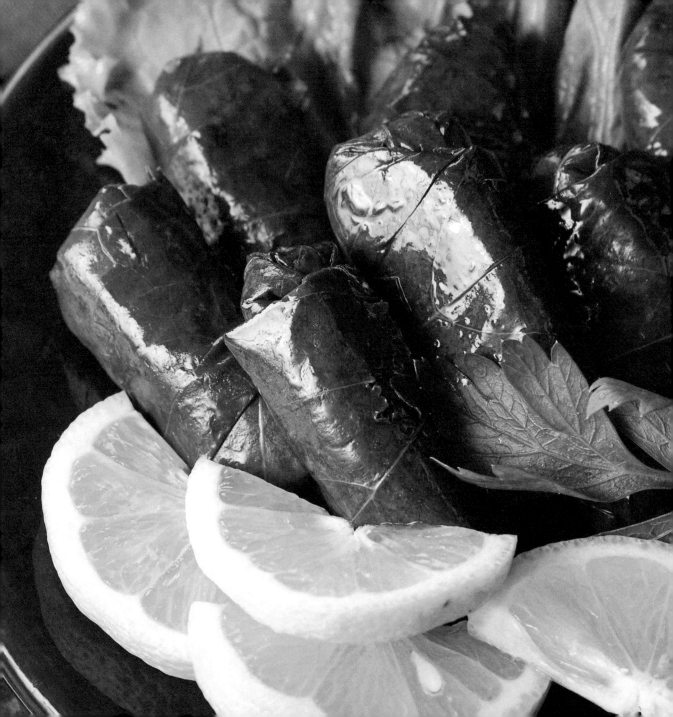

Wash leaves and stack them in a bowl. Dissolve salt in water, add whey/culture, and pour this liquid over the grape leaves. Place a smaller bowl or plate on top of the grape leaves to weigh them down so they remain submerged in the liquid. Cover the bowl with a cheesecloth or napkin, set aside, and let the leaves ferment for 3 days. Then transfer the leaves carefully into a pint jar, fill this (to one inch below the top) with the liquid, cover it with the lid, and refrigerate for up to one week.

Step two: Rice Filling

- 2 cups water, plus more if needed
- 1 cup brown rice
- 1 onion, chopped
- ½ cup parsley, chopped
- 2 bay leaves
- 2 cloves garlic, crushed
- 3 lemons, cut in half and seeded
- 2 tablespoons tomato paste
- 2 tablespoons olive oil
- ½ stick celery
- ¼ cup mint, chopped
- 1 tablespoon dried dill
- ½ teaspoon cumin

- ½ teaspoon paprika
- ¼ cup yogurt
- Optional: ½ cup pine nuts or chopped almonds, ¼ cup dried currants or raisins, ¼ cup chopped kalamata olives

Sauté onion, garlic, and celery in olive oil at bottom of stockpot or soup pot. Add rice, water, and all other ingredients except for yogurt. Cover this, bring it to a boil, then reduce to a simmer until rice is soft, about 30–45 minutes. Once rice is cooked, remove from heat and cool it to room temperature, then mix in yogurt. Taste the rice mixture and adjust it to your preferences by adding additional yogurt, lemon juice, or sea salt.

Finally, spread out fermented grape leaves on a cutting board or baking sheet. Fill each one with some of the rice mixture, leaving some empty space on each side. Fold up the top and bottom of the grape leaf first, bending each end back as well as you can. Then fold the sides over these, wrapping up the filling as tightly as possible. Turn over each dolma so that these ends are tucked underneath it, helping to secure them in place. You can eat or refrigerate these immediately or let them ferment at room temperature for a few hours longer before enjoying them.

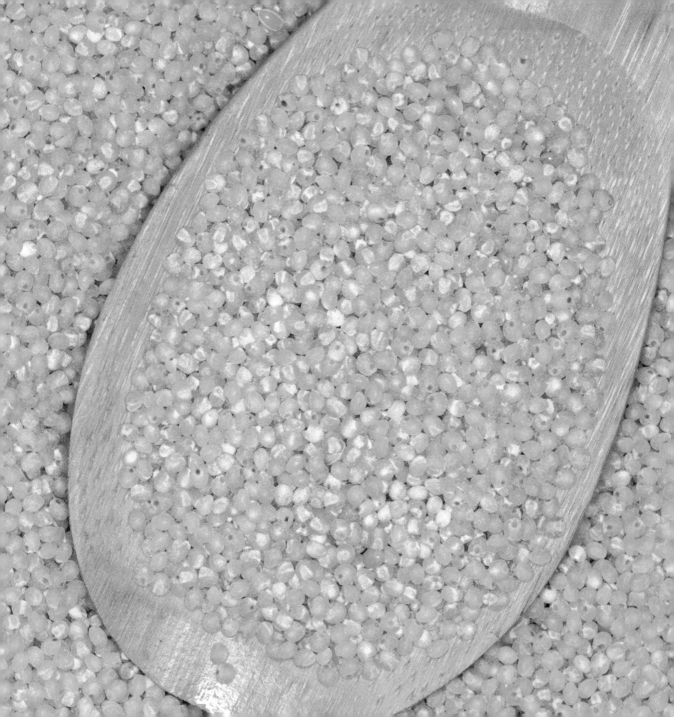

African Millet Beverage
(Koko in Ghana or Kunu in Nigeria)

Makes about 2 cups

Koko can be prepared as a drink or a porridge. Traditionally, the raw liquid portion of this is boiled, then cooled, and mixed with the raw, cultured solids to make a fermented gruel or porridge, sometimes called koko or ogi. Feel free to try this as well: I prefer to drink the liquid and feed the solids to the chickens, but perhaps you like spiced millet more than I do! There are many variations of this in West and Central Africa. This is a slightly simplified recipe.

* 2 cups water
* 1 cup CRASH milk, preferably almond milk
* ½ cup millet or sorghum grain
* 1 tablespoon yogurt whey or water kefir
* 1 inch ginger root, peeled and finely chopped
* ¼ teaspoon ground cloves
* ¼ teaspoon cardamom
* ¼ teaspoon cinnamon
* ½ teaspoon sea salt
* ⅛ teaspoon each: cayenne pepper and black pepper
* Honey, sugar, or maple syrup, to taste

Soak millet in water for 8–12 hours. Grind or crush in food processor or by using mortar and pestle. Add spices and salt. Move to jar, container, or pot and cover with water. Cover container and let it ferment at room temperature for 2–3 hours. Pour liquid into a glass, add sweetener to taste, and enjoy.

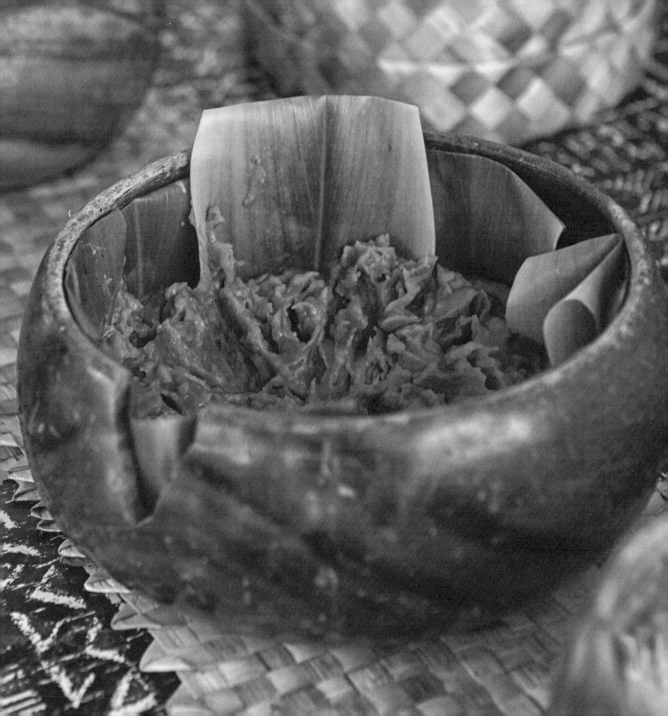

Poi (Hawaiian Fermented Taro)

Poi, the traditional Hawaiian and Polynesian dish, consists of taro corms or tubers. These are boiled, mashed, and then lactofermented. Poi has a sour flavor that is rather like sourdough. Try eating it with other foods such as meat, fish, beans, vegetables, or other starches.

Traditionally, Polynesians make poi by boiling and peeling taro corms or tubers, mashing them, adding a little water, and then letting it sit for 2–3 days to ferment naturally. You can buy taro roots in the grocery section of most Asian and Latin American food markets. As with other lactofermented foods, you can choose to add some yogurt whey or water kefir for a faster probiotic fermentation, or else just leave it a little longer and let the naturally present bacteria and yeasts ferment it themselves.

- ½ pound taro tubers (or corms)
- Water, as needed
- Optional: yogurt whey, sauerkraut juice, water kefir, or vegetable culture

Wash the taro. Put the tubers in a pot and add enough water to cover them. Cover pot with lid and put it on the stove on high heat. Bring to a boil, then turn down to medium heat. Cook until taro is soft enough that you can stick a fork through it. Pour out water over a colander, straining out the taro. Run some cold water over the taro to cool it. When it is cool enough to touch, gently peel off the skins. Place peeled taro tubers in a bowl or use a mortar and pestle. Mash them using a potato masher or large fork if they are in a bowl. Add a little water to the taro, continuing to mash and mix until it becomes a thin paste. Then mix in any culture you plan to use, cover the taro paste loosely, and allow it to ferment. Taste it after 24 hours and move it to the refrigerator as soon as it is sour enough for you, probably 1–4 days. Poi should last for a couple of weeks in the refrigerator.

Hummus

Makes about 2 cups

This wonderful Middle Eastern spread can anchor a variety of snacks or meals. It has been one of my family's favorites for many years, and I am glad to see how popular it has become. We normally spread hummus on pita bread, make sandwiches with it, or use it as a dip for vegetable sticks or chips. You can add many additional flavorings to this basic recipe, such as roasted red peppers, olives, or pine nuts. You can cut out the oil for a lower-calorie version—just use a little extra liquid (water, kefir, or yogurt whey) to achieve the consistency you need.

For the creamiest hummus, you will need to either peel the beans (which is tedious) or purée them when they are still very hot from being cooked. If you use canned beans, then heat them up first. Once they are cold, the skin gets too hard to purée them in a food processor and the hummus stays chunkier. One final option is to strain the hummus purée through a tight mesh strainer to remove the pieces of bean skin. I find this step to be more trouble than it is worth, but you are welcome to try it.

- 2 cups garbanzo beans (chickpeas), cooked
- ¼ cup tahini or 1 tablespoon sesame oil
- 2–3 tablespoons olive oil
- Juice of 1–3 lemons (about ¼ cup to ½ cup lemon juice), depending on your taste preference
- 2 cloves garlic
- 2 tablespoons parsley, chopped
- 2 tablespoons yogurt
- 1 teaspoon paprika
- 1 teaspoon sea salt
- ½ teaspoon cumin
- Pinch of black pepper
- Additional water as needed

Purée all ingredients in a food processor. Put the hummus in a container, cover it loosely, and allow it to ferment for 8–12 hours. Then cover it and place in the refrigerator, where it will last for 1–2 weeks. If you wish, reserve some paprika to sprinkle on top before serving.

Egg Salad with Sauerkraut or Pickles

Makes 3–4 servings

This makes a tangy egg salad spread, which is great on bread, crackers, and vegetable sticks (like carrot and celery sticks).

To make hard-boiled eggs, place a pot of water on the stove, and put your eggs inside it. Bring it to a boil, turn down the heat until it is a low boil, and let the eggs cook for 10 minutes. Take them out and rinse in cold water immediately to cool. Peel the eggs and rinse off any remaining pieces of shell. Older eggs are easier to peel than fresher ones.

Chop the hardboiled eggs. In a bowl, combine them with other ingredients and season to taste.

- ½ dozen large eggs, hard-boiled and shelled
- ½ stick celery, finely chopped
- ¼ cup sauerkraut or natural pickles, finely chopped
- ½ teaspoon garlic powder or small clove of fresh garlic, crushed
- 1 teaspoon mustard or mustard powder
- Mayonnaise or yogurt, to taste
- Salt and pepper, to taste

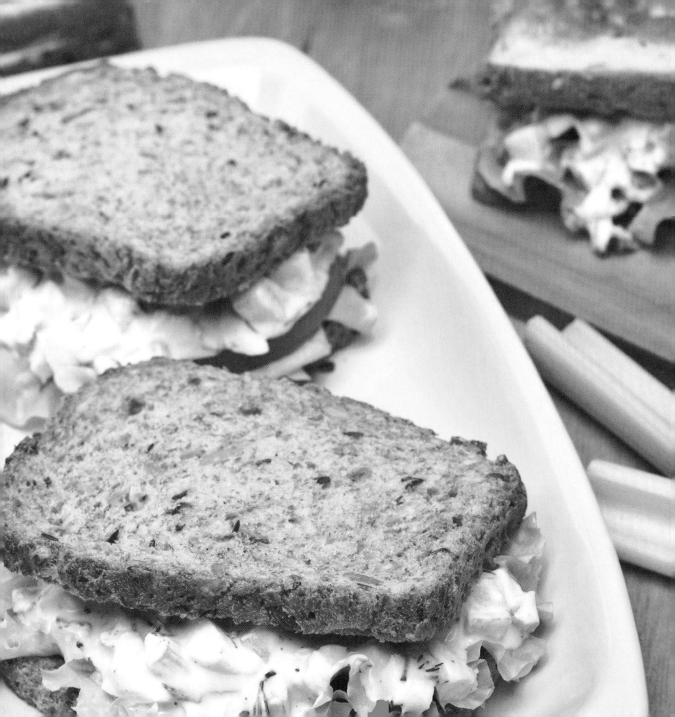

Purple Pickled Eggs

Makes 6 pickled eggs

Pickled eggs are a traditional dish in German, Eastern European, and Jewish cuisines. These cultures have deep pickling traditions—they seem to pickle nearly everything. Though almost anything can be pickled using natural lactofermentation, eggs are one of the more difficult foods to ferment this way. Why? There just isn't that much ready fuel in eggs for the probiotic organisms. This means they get off to a slower start than they do when you introduce them to the natural sugars of milk, grains, vegetables, or fruits. And slow starts can spell trouble because they leave an opening for molds.

This recipe addresses the problem by submerging hard-boiled eggs in probiotic-cultured brine such as pickle juice. If there's no open air under the brine, then mold cannot grow there. And it does not really matter whether the eggs themselves get fermented because they will be pickled in probiotic brine anyway. One way or another, they will taste pickled, they will be teeming with probiotics, and they can be safely consumed, which are the three goals of this recipe. The purple color comes from adding beets.

First, you need to create a brine. For this, you can follow the recipe for Naturally Cultured Pickles or for Dilly Beans and Carrot Sticks just using the water and flavoring ingredients but not the main vegetables (the cucumbers, beans, etc.) in those recipes. It is best to have the brine already fermented by the time you combine it with the eggs, giving them the quickest start possible. You will need enough pickling brine to fill one or two large Mason jars or other containers.

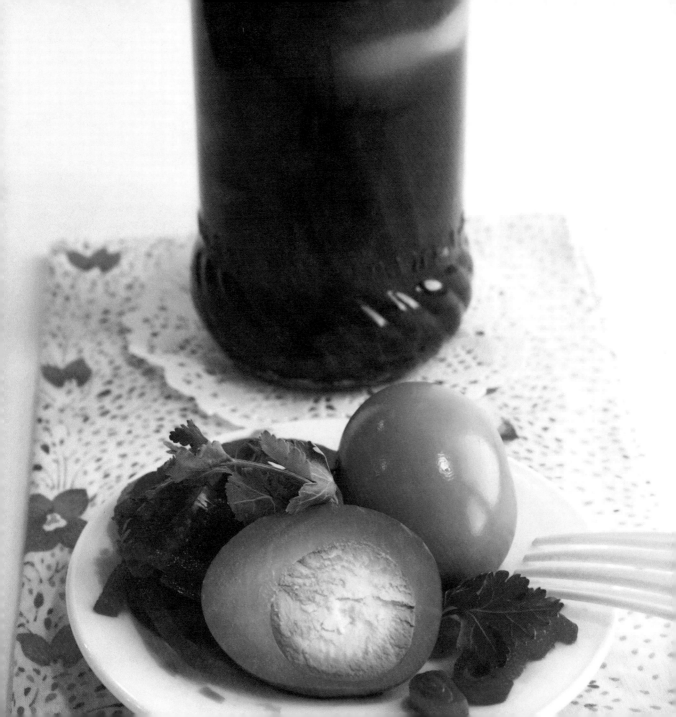

- 6 hard-boiled eggs (see page 90)
- ½ cup beets, peeled and sliced (cooked or raw)
- ½ cup sliced onion
- 1 pint to 1 quart pickle juice or probiotic brine (from Naturally Cultured Pickles or for Dilly Beans and Sticks recipe)
- Sea salt, to taste, if pickle brine is not used

Place hard-boiled eggs and vegetables in jars or containers. Leave a few inches of space at the top since the probiotic culture must cover eggs completely. If needed, weigh them down with a cheese weight, a stone that is food-safe, or a smaller container that is filled with water. Let them ferment for 1–2 days, making sure the eggs remain submerged in the brine.

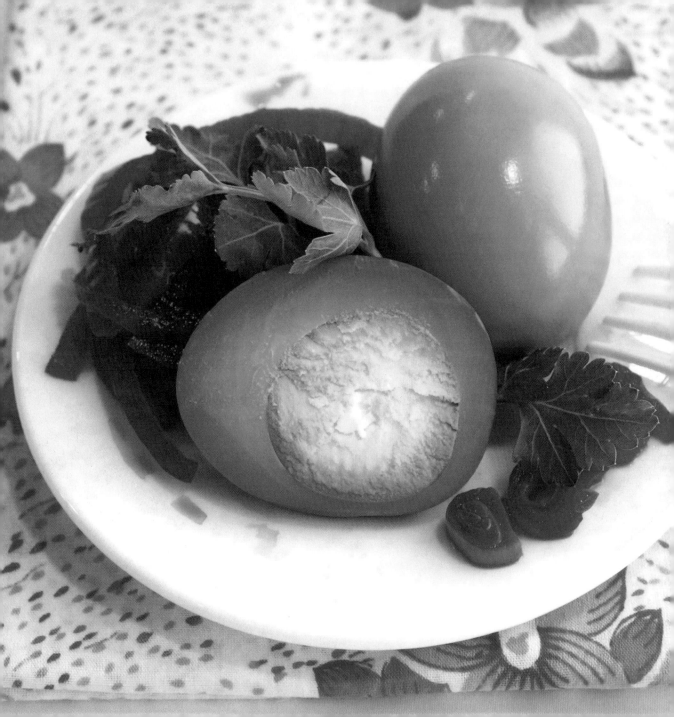

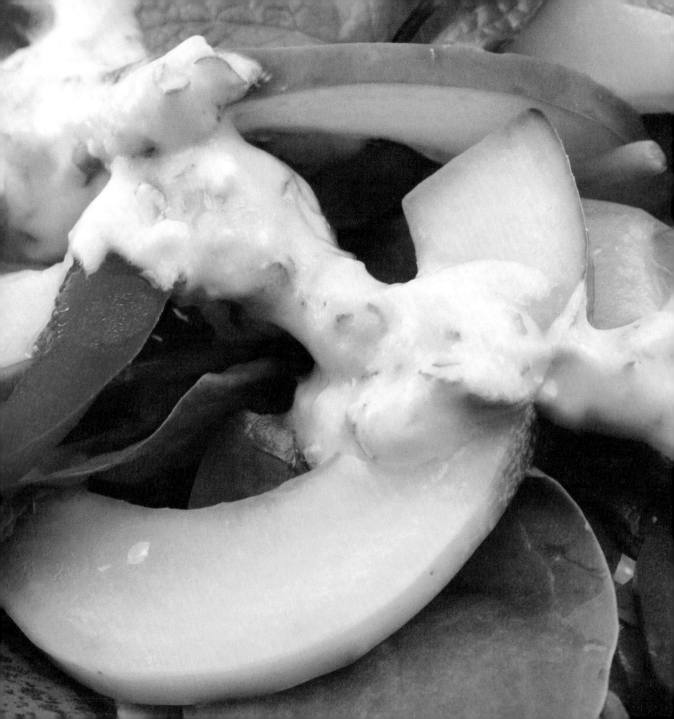

Chapter 10
Fermented Condiments, Salad Dressing, Jam, and Chutney

In Western cuisine, many of the sour flavors we are accustomed to come from our condiments and salad dressings. If you enjoy eating sandwiches, burgers, and salads, then adding a cultured condiment or dressing provides a great way to get your probiotics. Of course, you also can add a natural pickle or some sauerkraut, chutney, guacamole, or corn salsa (see separate recipes) for an even greater benefit. This chapter also covers one recipe each for a probiotic jam and chutney.

The condiment recipes for probiotic mayonnaise, ketchup, garlic mustard, yogurt chive salad dressing, and kombucha vinaigrette salad dressing become probiotic when you add yogurt, kefir, or sauerkraut juice to them. If you wish, you can also let them ferment at room temperature. This creates a stronger sour flavor and increases the probiotic content.

Mayonnaise

Makes about 2 cups

- 3 egg yolks, allowed to warm for a few minutes at room temperature
- 1½ cups olive oil, plus more if needed (may substitute with another oil)
- ¼ cup lemon juice

- 3 tablespoons yogurt or kefir (or 2 tablespoons sauerkraut juice)
- ¼ teaspoon onion powder
- ¼ teaspoon mustard powder
- ¼ teaspoon sea salt, plus more to taste (you may not need any if you use sauerkraut juice)

Blend egg yolks, half the lemon juice, mustard and onion powders, and sea salt. Open blender lid and begin to add the olive oil *very* slowly as the blender runs. Pace yourself so that it takes at least 3 minutes to add all the olive oil; this is how slow you need to pour it or drip it in. The oil will only get incorporated into the emulsion if you add it at a slow stream. Add only as much oil as you need to get the right thickness for your mayonnaise, keeping it a little too thick if you are using sauerkraut juice. Finally, add the yogurt, kefir, or sauerkraut juice. Taste and add additional sea salt or lemon juice if needed. Turn off the blender, scrape out the mayonnaise into a bowl or container, and enjoy. Lasts about one week in the refrigerator.

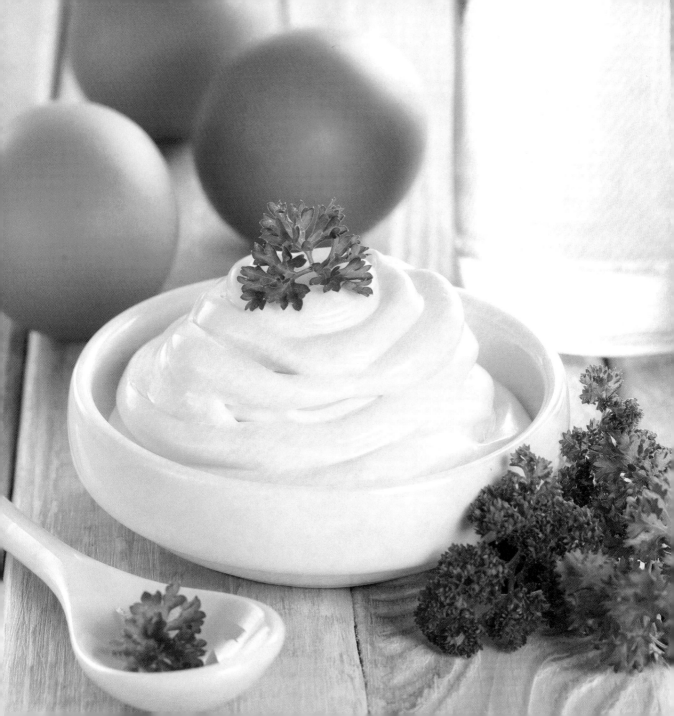

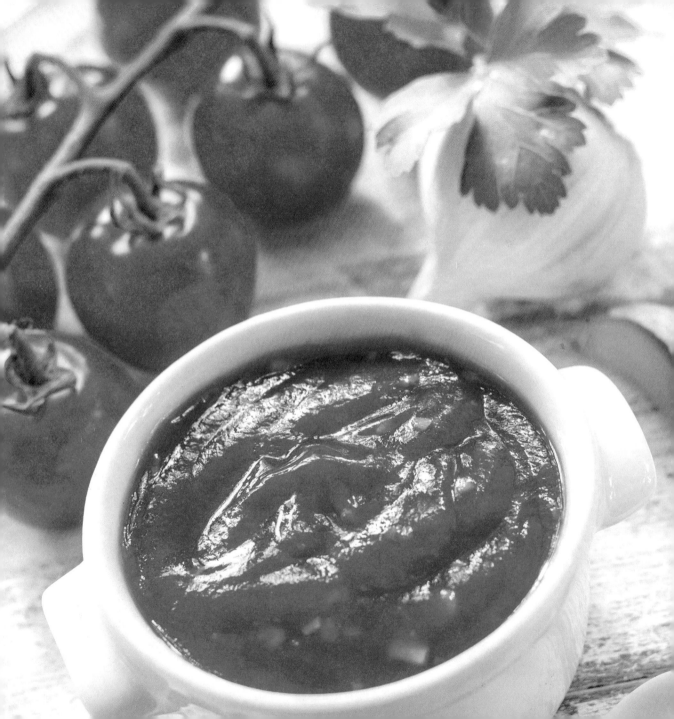

Ketchup

Makes about 2½ cups

- 2 cups tomato paste
- ¼ cup maple syrup, honey, or brown sugar
- ¼ cup yogurt, kefir, or sauerkraut juice
- 2 tablespoons apple cider vinegar
- 1 teaspoon lemon juice, plus zest of half a lemon
- 1 teaspoon sea salt, plus more to taste (you may not need any if you use sauerkraut juice)
- 1 teaspoon allspice
- ½ teaspoon onion powder
- ¼ teaspoon mustard powder
- ¼ teaspoon ground cloves
- Optional: one small clove garlic (crushed) or small handful chives (diced)

Thoroughly mix together all ingredients in a mixing bowl or a blender. Taste and make any needed adjustments to suit your preferences, adding extra sea salt, spices, or lemon juice. Transfer to a jar or container to store in the refrigerator or ferment at room temperature for up to 3–5 days. This will keep in the fridge for at least two weeks.

Garlic Mustard

Makes about 2 cups

- 1¼ cups brown mustard seeds (may substitute up to half with black mustard seeds, which are spicier)
- ½ cup water, plus 3 cups for soaking seeds
- ¼ cup lemon juice
- 1–2 cloves garlic, crushed
- 3 tablespoons yogurt, kefir, or sauerkraut juice
- 2 teaspoons maple syrup, honey, or brown sugar
- 1 teaspoon turmeric powder
- 1 teaspoon sea salt, plus more to taste (you may not need any if you use sauerkraut juice)
- 1 tablespoon sea salt for soaking seeds
- ½ teaspoon onion powder

Wash the mustard seeds. Place them in a bowl or jar with 1 tablespoon salt, cover with 3 cups of water, and let the seeds soak in this salt water for 24–48 hours. Drain them using a strainer. Grind with a mortar and pestle, blender, or food processor. For whole grain mustard, crush only half of the seeds. Mix in the other ingredients, taste, and add additional salt or spices if you prefer. For a really smooth mustard, you can run it through a strainer to remove any hulls. Transfer mustard into a jar or container, cover loosely, and let it ferment at room temperature for 2–3 days before moving to the refrigerator. It will last for at least two weeks in the fridge.

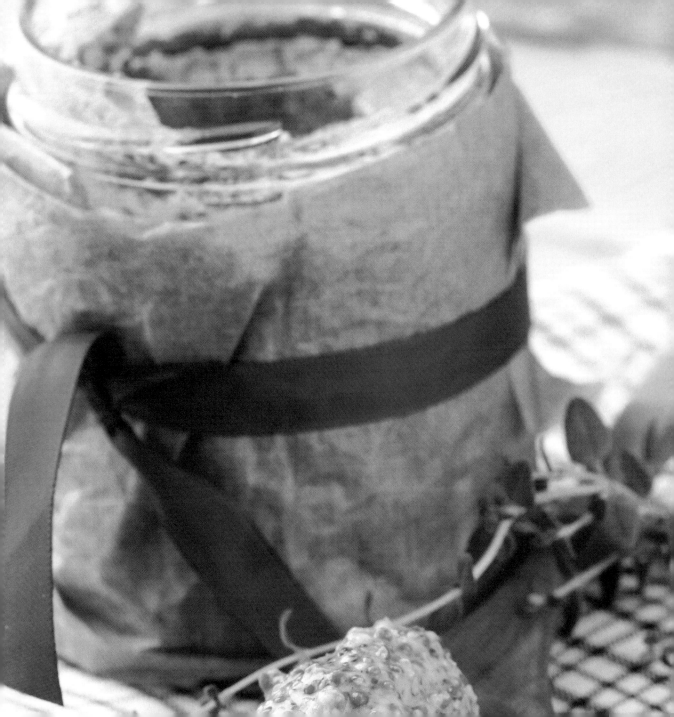

Yogurt Chive Salad Dressing

Makes ½ cup of salad dressing, about enough to dress one large salad

- ¼ cup yogurt
- 2 tablespoons chives, finely chopped
- 1 tablespoon parsley, finely chopped
- Juice and zest of half a lemon
- 1 tablespoon olive oil
- ¼ teaspoon sugar or honey
- ¼ teaspoon sea salt
- Dash of black pepper or cayenne pepper

Mix together all ingredients in a bowl or a blender. I like the taste of fresh herbs, so I do not ferment this dressing, but you can leave it at room temperature for a few hours if you wish.

Kombucha Vinaigrette Salad Dressing

Makes ½ cup of salad dressing, about enough to dress one large salad

- ¼ cup kombucha
- ¼ cup olive oil, or more if you prefer
- 1 tablespoon lemon juice
- 1 teaspoon fresh herbs (chopped finely), such as thyme, marjoram, oregano, tarragon and/or rosemary
- ½ teaspoon garlic powder
- ½ teaspoon onion powder
- ½ teaspoon maple syrup, honey, or brown sugar
- Dash of black pepper
- Optional: Replace onion and garlic powder with 1 clove garlic (crushed) or ¼ cup red onion or shallot, diced

Mix together all ingredients using a blender. Taste and adjust flavor by adding additional oil, salt, or lemon juice as necessary. The major variation with this one is the strength of the kombucha, which can be mild (requiring more lemon juice) or very vinegary (perhaps requiring more oil). I like the taste of fresh herbs, so I do not ferment this dressing, but you can leave it at room temperature for a few hours if you wish.

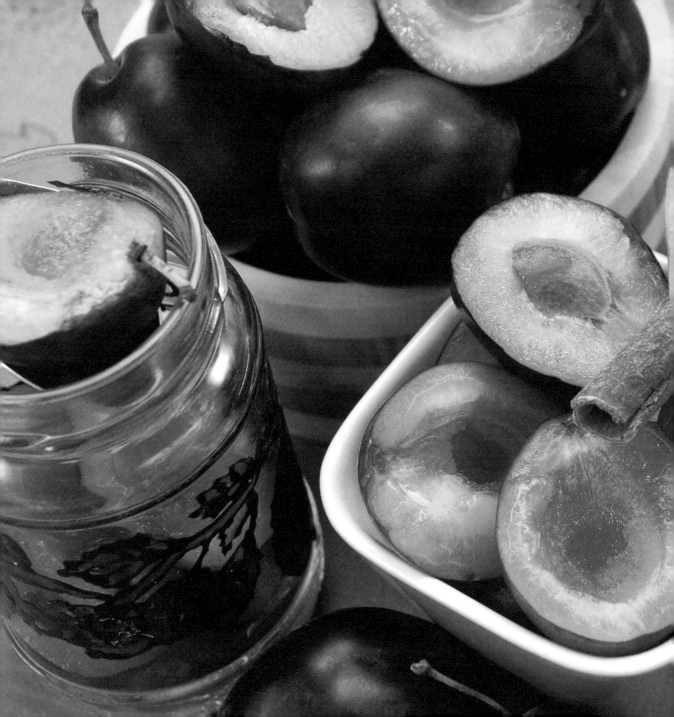

Plum Ginger Jam

Makes 3–4 cups

Jam ingredients:

- 2 pounds ripe plums, pitted and chopped
- ½ cup gingery honey (recipe below; takes 5 days)
- ½ teaspoon sea salt
- Optional: 2 tablespoons yogurt whey, water kefir, cider, or other culture

Gingery honey:

- 1 inch piece of ginger, peeled and finely chopped
- ½ cup honey

Put chopped ginger in a jar or cup. Cover with honey. After 5 days, mix it together and use honey.

To make the jam, start with a mixing bowl. Combine plums, gingery honey, salt, and the optional culture. Stir these together, then transfer to a jar or container. Let it ferment for 3 days and then transfer to refrigerator. You can use right away and as needed; it will keep in the refrigerator for about one month.

Curried Apple Chutney

Makes about 6 cups

This is a tasty side dish that you can enjoy with just about any main course. Choose a firm variety of apple, such as Granny Smith, Rome Beauty, Honeycrisp, Golden Delicious, Empire, Northern Spy, or Pink Lady. If you prefer, you can substitute firm peaches or pears instead of apples.

- 6 cups sliced apples (apple pie size)
- ½ cup whey or water kefir
- ½ cup lemon juice
- ¼ cup sugar (or more, to taste)
- 1 teaspoon sea salt
- 4 teaspoons mild curry powder
- Optional: 1 cup raisins, 1 cup chopped celery, or 1 cup sliced green bell pepper (each provide an additional sweet or savory taste)

Mix all ingredients in a bowl and taste to ensure the proportions are about right for you (add more of anything as needed). Transfer to a jar, crock, or other container, and cover loosely. You may like this a little sweet or with a stronger sour taste; start tasting it after one day and be prepared to give it 2–4 days to ferment. Once it is ready, cover the container tightly and store it in the refrigerator for up to two weeks.

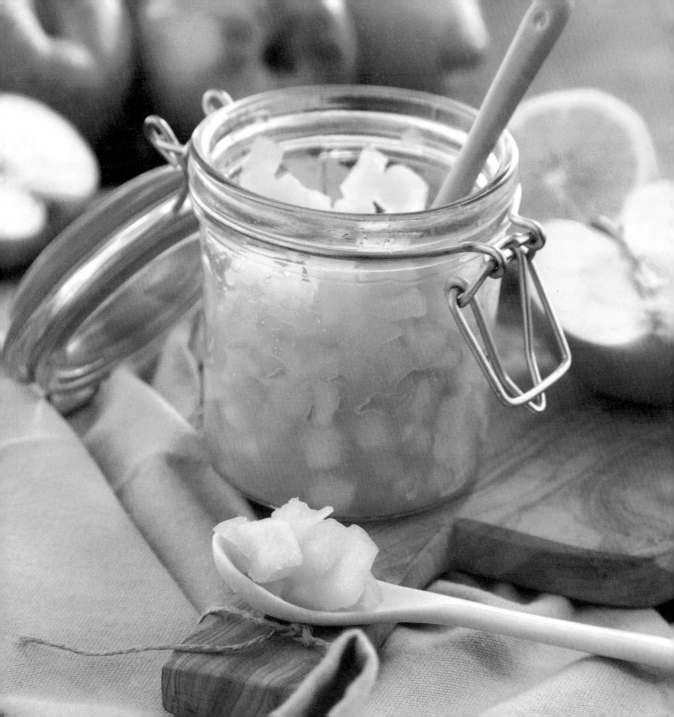

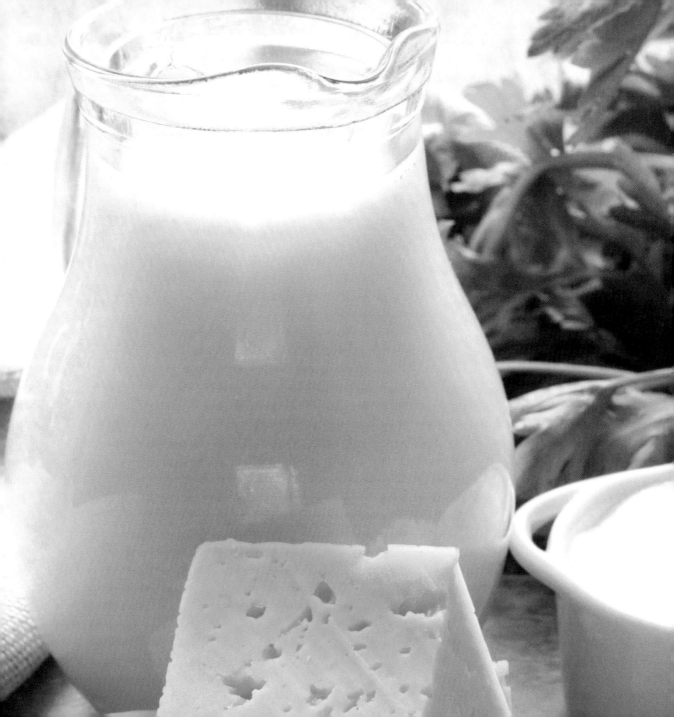

Chapter 11
Simple Cultured Cheeses

Cheese is one of the great fermented foods of the world, yet many of us do not think of it as being probiotic. This is because most store-bought cheese is no longer a live food; its culturing process has been halted to help preserve it. Also, some people think all cheese is fermented by molds (like blue cheese), even though probiotic bacterial cultures are used frequently. Even so, adding the starter culture (filled with good bacteria) is one of the first steps in a long process. Starter cultures are mainly used for flavoring and their main work is done in a matter of hours.

Can this beneficial bacteria make it all the way through the cheese-making process and end up in the final product you consume? The answer is yes, particularly with certain fresh and aged cheeses. Raw, aged gouda, cheddar, and Parmegiano-Reggiano cheeses have been found to contain beneficial lactobacteria. Soft cheeses, such as cottage cheese, feta, and chevre (goat cheese) are even easier to culture and make at home. You will need a few basic supplies and ingredients, such as cheese starter cultures, rennet, calcium chloride, cheese moulds (not molds), and (if you wish) some cheese wax for aged cheeses, all of which are available at many health food stores and online from cheese-making supply stores.

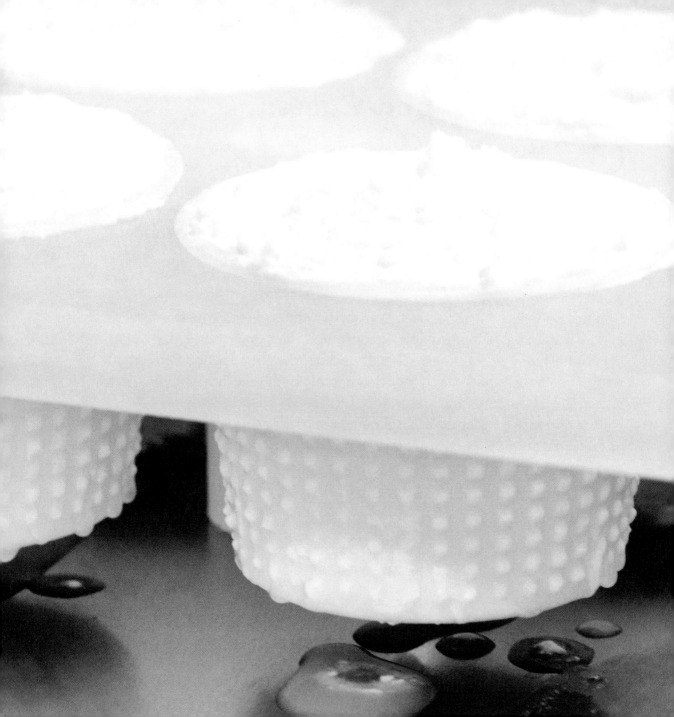

Surprisingly, cheese may be one of the best probiotic foods in the world. Studies have demonstrated that because of cheese's protein and fat complex, and the way our bodies digest this, cheese is extremely effective at delivering probiotic cultures deep into our digestive systems. With some other foods, the cultures are broken down in the stomach, so these cultures never have a chance to colonize in our guts. Apparently, cheese allows them to make it further down. Bottom line: eating probiotic cheese may be one of the best ways to rebuild and maintain your body's probiotic health.

The recipes below cover cottage, feta, chevre (soft goat cheese), and gouda cheeses. They are probably the most difficult recipes in this book. I chose them both because of their probiotic benefits and because these are some of the simpler cheeses to make. Best of luck!

Cottage Cheese

Makes about 4 cups

Most cottage cheese recipes involve cooking the curds above 110°F, which does not help their probiotic content. This recipe uses a two-stage culturing process to create a live, active-cultured cottage cheese. First, mesophilic starter culture or buttermilk is used to separate the curd from the whey and create the proper flavor. After the curds are cut, drained, cooked, and drained again, yogurt whey or kefir adds a strong probiotic culture. Yes, you can use buttermilk as a source of culture for this cheese if you want, though the curd size will be smaller.

- 1 gallon milk (cow or goat milk)
- 1 package mesophilic direct-set cheese starter culture *or* ½ cup cultured buttermilk
- ½ rennet tablet (or ½ teaspoon liquid rennet), dissolved in ¼ cup water
- 2 tablespoons yogurt whey or kefir
- Optional: ½ teaspoon to 1 teaspoon sea salt

In a large pot, using a cheese thermometer, heat milk to 75°F. Add a culture packet or buttermilk, stir it in, and cover. The culture will take about 24 hours to do its job. During this time, its ideal temperature is 70–75°F, so try to insulate the pan if your air temperature is lower than this. Consider putting some warm water bottles around the pan and covering it with a towel or two, for example.

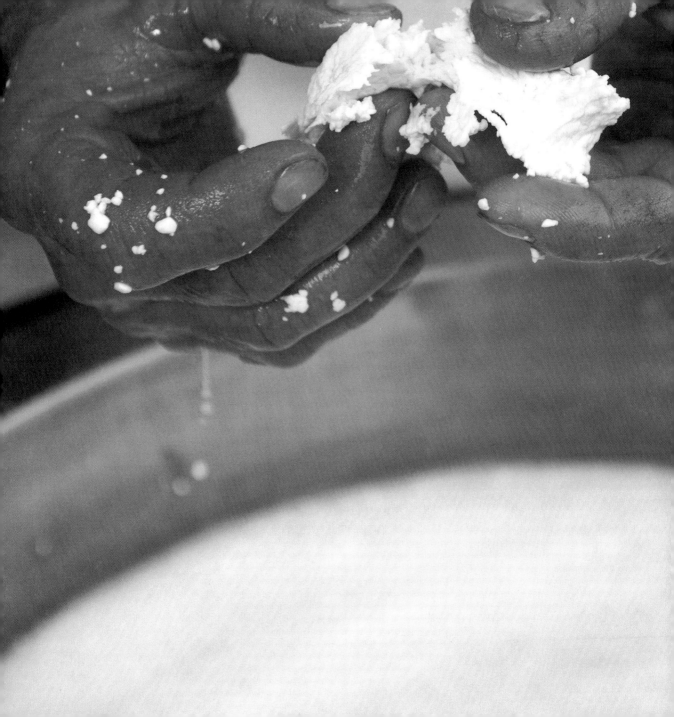

After 24 hours, the curd should be thick. Using a long knife, cut it horizontally and vertically (like a grid) to make ½-inch cubes. Then, let the curds sit for 15 minutes as you get the hot water bath ready.

Next, you need to heat the curds to 110–120°F. The easiest way to do this is to place the pot of curds in a water bath. Fill up a large sink, basin, or bathtub with really hot water, slightly above the level of the curds in the pot. Conveniently, if we turn our tap to hot water, it comes out at 120°F. If yours is cooler, then you may need to boil a pot or two and dump it in also.

You need to hold the water temperature in this hot range for 25 minutes, which may require adding additional hot water, possibly after draining out a little cooler stuff. Stir the curds gently, once every 5 minutes. When the curds look like they have both shrunken and firmed up, you can stop the water bath and strain out the curds from the whey. The easiest methods are to use a strainer, a colander lined with cheesecloth, or a straining bag.

As the curds drain, wash them with cold water over the sink to bring down their temperature to no more than 50°F. If you prefer, you can move the colander/strainer/bag to a bath of ice water to chill them. Then strain and drain curd again. Once drained, which can take 30–60 minutes, you are finished with the difficult part. Before placing cheese in the refrigerator, add sea salt and whey/kefir. Stir this in, cover the cottage cheese, and move it to the refrigerator. You can eat it any time for the next two weeks or so.

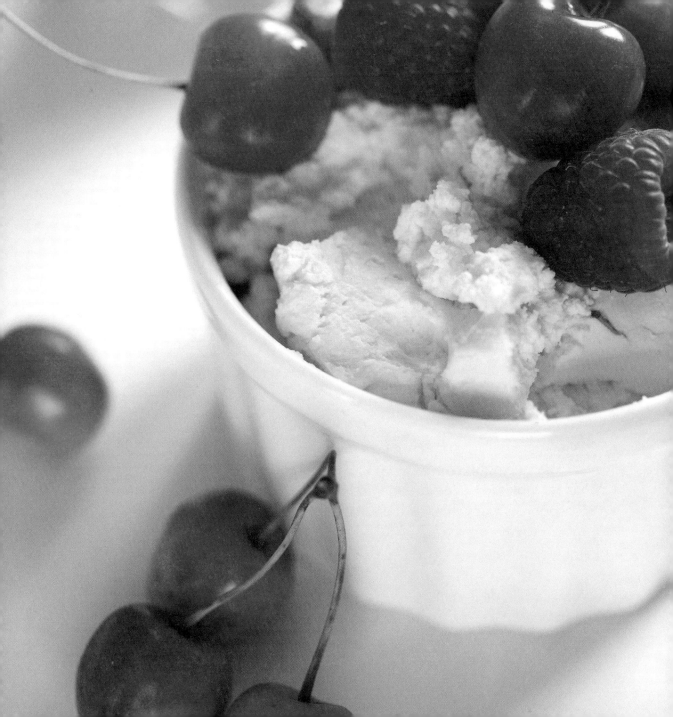

Feta Cheese

Makes 1 pound

This recipe uses yogurt as a cheese culture. I have adapted it from the *Cultures for Health* website, which is located at www.culturesforhealth.com and is an excellent source of fermentation supplies. To make the cheese set properly, you also will need calcium chloride and rennet (regular, vegetable, or microbial). The calcium chloride is optional, but highly recommended. Most milk is lacking in calcium, especially if it has been processed, and adding additional calcium ensures the cheese will set. You can get both rennet and calcium chloride at health food stores or online at a chef's or cheese-making supply store. Use a large stainless steel or nonmetal pot, since cheese ingredients may react with other metals. Nonmetal containers are best for the cultures also, but since few people have large nonmetal pots, stainless steel will do.

Primary ingredients:

- 1 gallon goat milk (you can use cow milk also)
- 1 tablespoon yogurt
- ½ rennet tablet (or ½ teaspoon liquid rennet), dissolved in ¼ cup water
- ⅛ teaspoon calcium chloride, dissolved in ¼ cup water

Ingredients for brine:

- ¼ cup sea salt, diluted in
- 2 quarts water

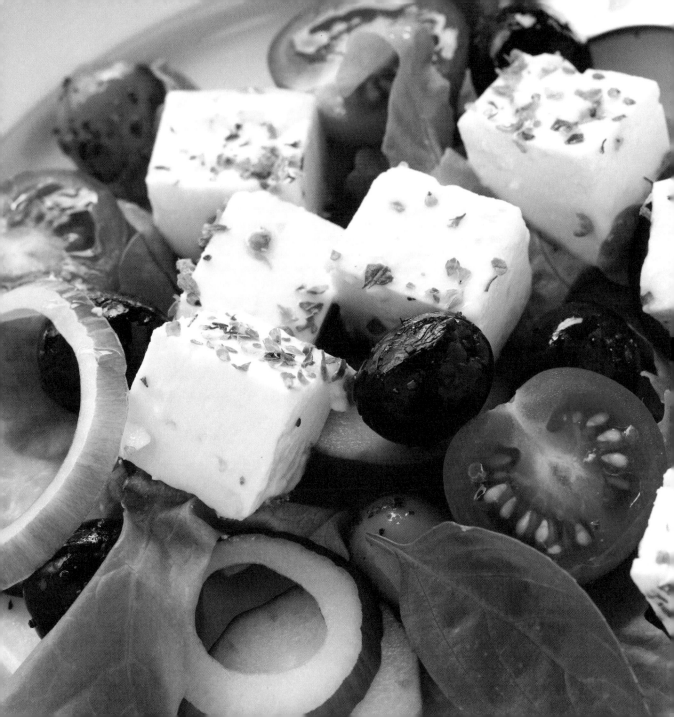

Dilute calcium chloride with ¼ cup water. In a large pot, using a cheese thermometer, heat milk to 86°F. As milk warms, add calcium-water solution to the milk and stir well. Once milk is partway to warm, take ½ cup of milk out, and mix yogurt into the ½ cup milk, crushing any lumps. At 86°F, take the pot off the heat, add the yogurt-milk culture, and stir it into the pot of milk. Cover loosely with a towel or cheesecloth. Let the cultured milk sit for 1 hour, at which time it should be room temperature.

With another ¼ cup of water, dilute the rennet. Add this to the cultured milk at room temperature and stir it *very lightly* with an up-down (not back-and-forth) motion of the spoon.

Cover the pot with a lid and let the cultured milk sit overnight (for 8–10 hours). When you check it again the next morning, there should be clear gelling and curd separation in the milk.

With a long knife, cut the curd into ½-inch cubes. Gently stir the curds for 20 minutes to complete their separation from the whey.

Pour out the contents of the pot over a colander or strainer lined with cheesecloth, separating the curds from the whey. Cover and let them continue to drain for 4 hours or until all liquid is gone (no more drips).

Place curds into a large jar or bowl and cover them with the salt brine solution. Let the curds brine for 4–5 days. At that point, you can begin eating the cheese. You can store the feta cheese cubes in this brine for up to one month.

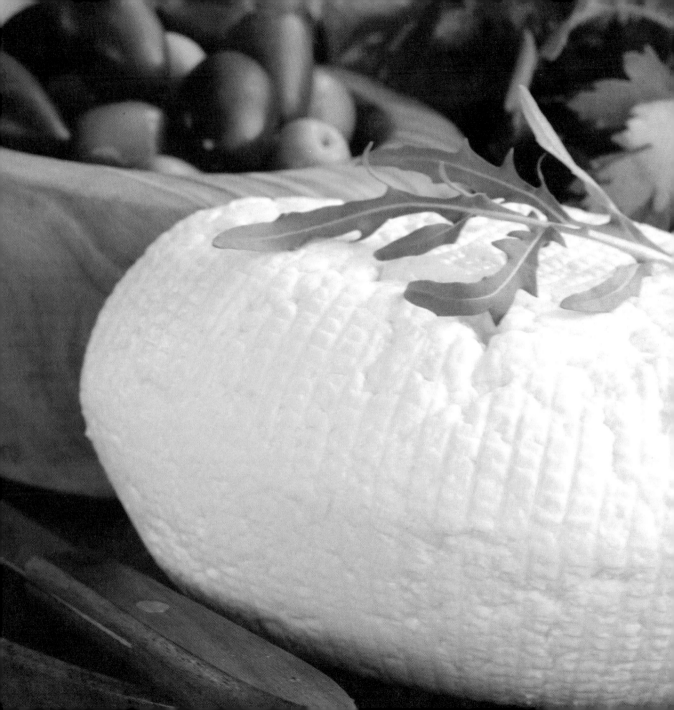

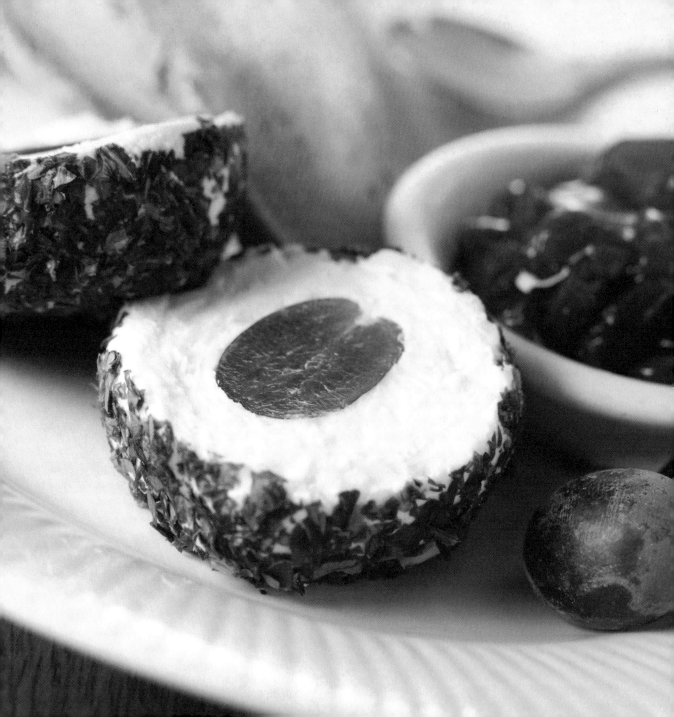

Chevre (Soft Goat Cheese)

Makes 1 pound

- 1 gallon goat milk (or use cow's milk for a cream cheese-style flavor)
- 1 package chevre culture
- Optional: 1 teaspoon yogurt whey or kefir

In a large pot, heat milk to 160°F, then cool to 86°F. Remove pot from heat and add chevre culture. Cover the pot and let it sit for 12 hours or until the cultured milk has the thickness of yogurt.

Optional: To introduce yogurt cultures, add the yogurt whey to the chevre curds and whey. Mix gently.

Strain and drain chevre over a strainer lined with tight cheesecloth or pour this into a straining bag. It will take 6–12 hours to drain the whey from the curds.

At this point, you can enjoy the fresh chevre as is, mix in some fresh or dried herbs, or ladle curds into chevre cheese moulds. Moulds are optional; you can purchase them online from cheese-making supply stores.

Cover moulds with plastic wrap or aluminum foil and put them in the refrigerator for 24–48 hours. You will need to put something under the moulds to catch any drippings. If you have a kitchen rack or food-safe screen, you can place the draining moulds on top of this, with a bowl or tray underneath. Alternatively, you can place them on a "block" above a tray or bowl. The "block" can be anything in the kitchen that fits and has a bit of flat surface, such as a cookie cutter, an overturned shot glass, or an overturned measuring cup. You just need something that will serve as a spacer, allowing any remaining liquid to drip down and keep it away from the curds in the mould.

For soft cheese like chevre, you do not need to place a weight on top of the mould—it will dry out and compact quite well by itself within a day or two.

Remove chevre from the mould by tapping it out. This is a great time to roll it in any flavoring if you choose to do so, such as dried or fresh herbs, garlic or onion powder, or edible ash (available online from cheese-making supply stores). Store your roll of chevre in plastic wrap or in a container. Delicious!

Gouda Cheese

Makes 1 pound

This recipe makes a baby gouda, which does not require aging. However, the flavor will improve if you age this cheese for 3–6 months.

- 1 gallon whole milk
- 1 package (⅛ teaspoon) Mesophilic M cheese culture
- ½ rennet tablet (or ½ teaspoon liquid rennet), dissolved in ¼ cup water
- ¼ teaspoon calcium chloride, dissolved in ¼ cup water
- Optional: 1 teaspoon yogurt whey or kefir

Heat milk to 90°F in a large stainless steel or nonmetal pot. Remove from heat, add Mesophilic M starter culture, and gently stir it in. Also add calcium-water solution.

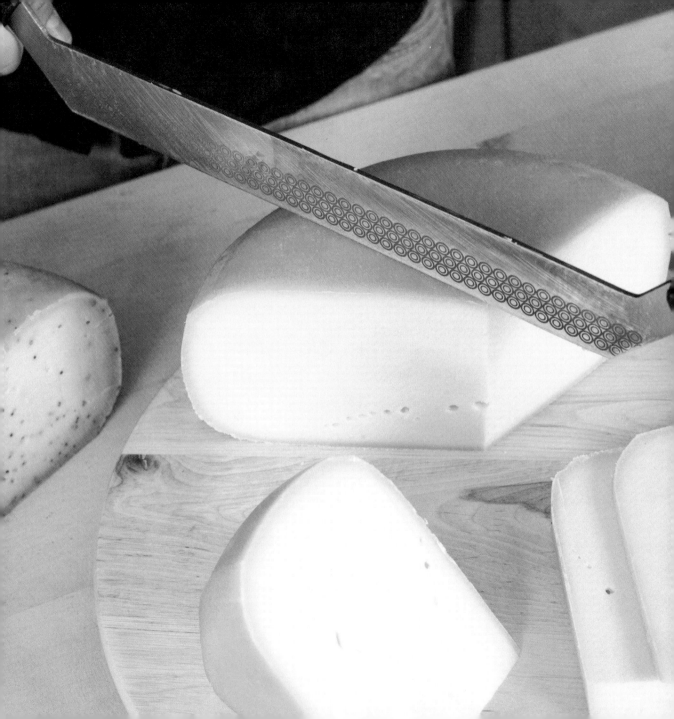

Then add rennet solution and mix this in gently for 1 minute with an up-down motion.

Let it sit for 1 hour or until curd has set. You can check for this by running a knife through the curd at an angle and picking up a little bit of the curd on the knife. If the curd breaks cleanly not sticking to the knife, and if the whey runs into the crack, then you have full separation. If you wait much longer, the curd will be too tough.

The next step is cutting the curd. The main reason to cut curd is to release the whey, which creates curds that will make a harder cheese. Your task is to cut the curd into 1–2-inch pieces, not much bigger or smaller. With the knife, cut vertical and horizontal columns so that each piece of curd is 1–2 inches on each side. Of course, getting the knife underneath them to make a clean bottom cut is a challenge, but luckily it is acceptable to cut at a 45-degree angle if needed. These pieces need not be cubic in shape.

Once you've cut off the top level of curds, use a spoon to pull up the bigger pieces and use the knife to cut them into 1–2-inch pieces. You may be able to use the spoon for this, but if it's not sharp enough, then use the knife. Stir the curds around to make sure you haven't left any; stirring for 3–5 minutes also helps ensure the curd is completely separated from the whey.

Let it settle for about 5 minutes. While waiting, bring a pot of water to 175°F. You will use this to raise the temperature of the curds. Add one cup of the hot water to the curds and gently stir curds for 10 minutes. Then let them settle for 10 more minutes, while you lower the temperature of the hot water pot to 150–170°F.

Using a strainer, colander, or some means of holding back the curds, pour off 4 cups of whey from the curd pot. Add four cups of hot water to the curd pot, replacing the whey. Stir it and check the temperature, which should be 100°F. You will need to keep it at 100°F for the next 20 minutes as you stir the curds. One way to do this is to fill sink a few inches high with 100–110°F water and place the pot in it.

After stirring for 20 minutes at 100°F, it is time to strain the curds from the whey. Use a strainer or colander lined with cheesecloth or a straining bag. First, make sure the curds are ready for straining by taking out a handful of them with a spoon, cooling them in cold water, and then squeezing them in your hand. If they stick together, you can strain the whole bunch. If not, wait 5 minutes before taking out the curds from the whey. Strain them, saving the whey or pouring it out. Then let the curds sit for 5 minutes before proceeding.

Optional: With the temperature coming down again, this is where you can add some more probiotic cultures if you choose. To do so, just drip the yogurt whey or kefir over the curds, mixing gently to distribute it.

While curds are still warm, put them into the cheese moulds and cover with the followers. Place 1-pound weights (or four rolls of pennies) on top of each mould for 15 minutes. Take cheese out and turn it over, covering again with followers, and this time pressing with 2–3 pounds for another 15 minutes.

Keep repeating this step with 2–3-pound pressure until the rind of the cheese is smooth without gaps. Then leave 2–3-pound weights on cheese overnight (for 8–10 hours).

Brine the cheese in a solution of 1½ cups salt diluted in ½ gallon of water. After pressing, place cheese in the brine and let this sit at room temperature for 2 hours. Air-dry the cheese on a rack or mat until it is dry to the touch. This can take up to one day.

To wax the cheese, melt some cheese wax (following the directions that come with the wax) and paint it on with a waxing brush, laying a thick coat all around the cheese. Then place it in the refrigerator and let the cheese age for 3–6 months.

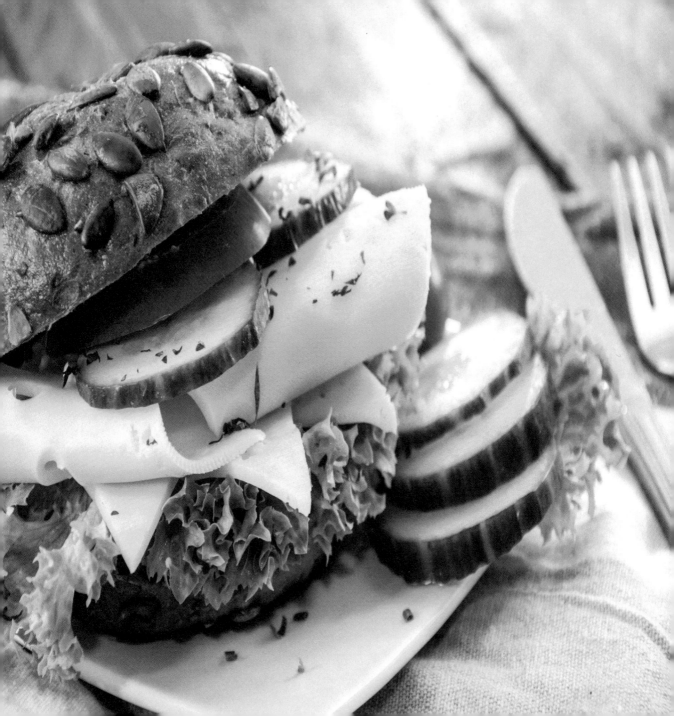

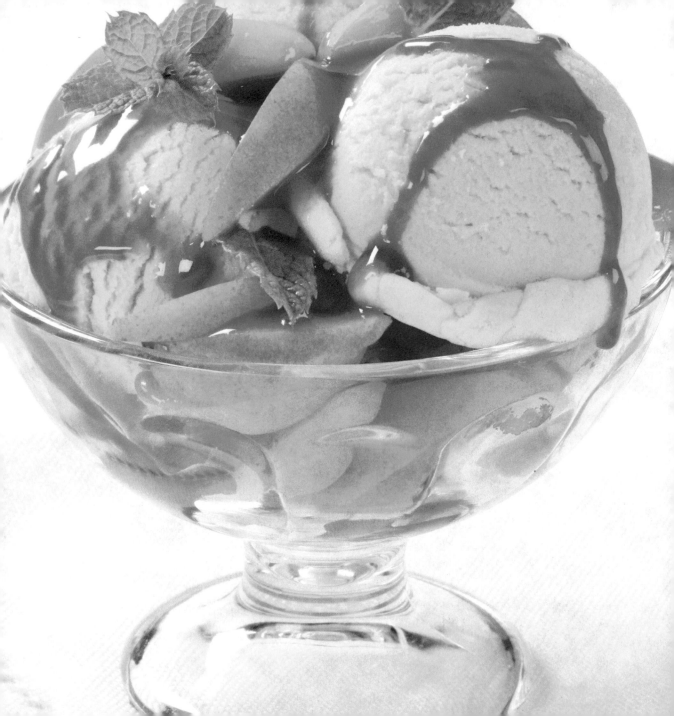

Chapter 12
Tasty Probiotic Desserts

In addition to the blended treats that appear in the chapter on smoothies and frozen desserts, there are many more ways to make probiotic desserts. The recipes in this chapter use yogurt, cottage cheese, kefir, or kombucha as main ingredients. You are welcome to add as much or as little sugar or sugar substitute as you wish. Aside from them all being probiotic, there is no other common thread between these desserts, so let's get right to the recipes!

Peach Ice Cream

Makes about 2 cups

You can make this refreshing ice cream alternative even without an ice cream maker. It's very low in fat and high in protein. Feel free to make it with other fruits instead of peaches. I made it with strawberries, which was delicious but quite sour (needing nearly two tablespoons of sugar). You control the sweetness by adding as much or as little sugar/sweetener as you wish, which will vary depending on the fruit and your tastes. My kids did not even guess there was cottage cheese in this!

- 1 cup cottage cheese
- 1 cup yogurt
- ½ cup milk or CRASH alternative
- 1½ cups sliced ripe peaches (or try substituting other fruit)
- 1 teaspoon vanilla extract, brandy, or peach liqueur

- Sugar, honey, or maple syrup (as needed)
- Optional: ¼ teaspoon cinnamon or ginger powder

Put all ingredients in a food processor or a good blender, then purée. Taste it and adjust sweetness by adding additional sugar, honey, or maple syrup as desired. Also, feel free to add a little more fruit if the taste is a bit bland.

If you have an ice cream machine, pour this mixture in and follow your ice cream machine's directions. If you do not have one, then pour the mixture into a container with a lid and freeze it. In 45–60 minutes, take out the container and stir the ice cream. Scrape the frozen parts off the edges and bottom and stir them into the middle. Then put it back in the freezer and repeat this procedure (checking, scraping the sides, and stirring) every 30 minutes.

Each time you do this, the ice cream will be thicker, and once it reaches the desired consistency, you can eat it. Depending on your freezer, you should have soft serve-style ice cream within about 90 minutes to 2 hours. At that point, it can become thick ice cream with one more 30-minute stir.

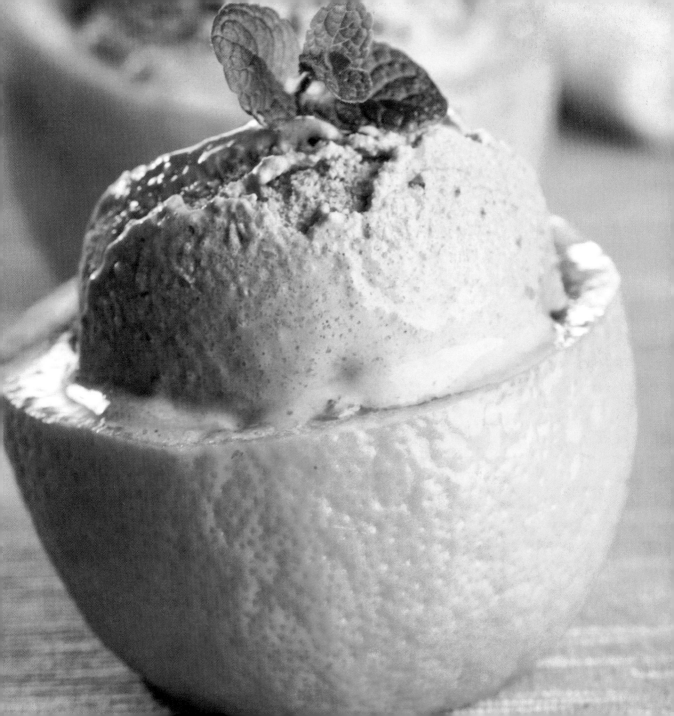

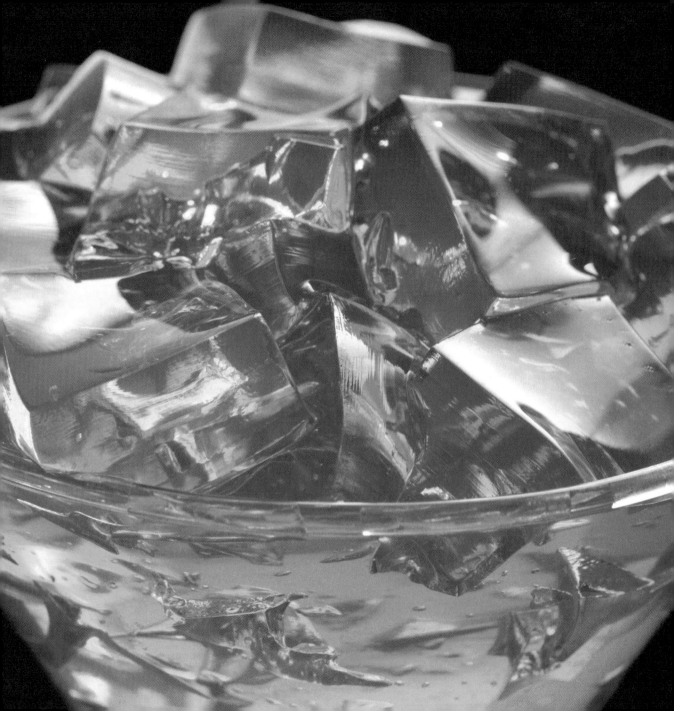

Kombucha Jelly Squares

Makes one 9 x 13 inch pan of jelly squares

If you like Jell-O™, then try making this probiotic alternative using kombucha, water kefir, or natural cider. You can make these squares in any flavor you wish. To keep the flavoring simple, this recipe incorporates one of the homemade soda syrups covered in this book (please see the chapter on making natural sodas for the recipes). Alternatively, you could use some maple syrup, chocolate syrup, or fruit jam. If you prefer a savory version, then skip the sweetener and try using some tomato juice, kale juice, or carrot juice, perhaps with a twist of lime and a little sea salt.

- 3 cups kombucha
- 1 cup homemade soda syrup (see chapter on making natural sodas for recipes)
- 1 tablespoon or more sugar, honey, maple syrup, or other sweetener
- 5 tablespoons gelatin or agar agar

Combine half of the kombucha in a pan with your soda syrup and sugar/sweetener. Follow directions on the package for your gelatin or agar agar, adding this to the sweetened/flavored kombucha, heating it, and stirring it as needed on the stove. As the mixture cools (again, following the gelatin or agar agar recipe on your package), add additional kombucha. Pour and spread on a baking sheet or jelly mould and let it cool. If you are using gelatin, you probably will need to cool this in the refrigerator, while the vegetarian alternative agar agar should firm up at room temperature. Once it is firm, cut the jelly into squares to serve.

Thanksgiving Cranberry-Orange Relish

Makes about 3 cups of relish

This autumn, relish may become a new classic in your kitchen. It's a great dish for Thanksgiving dinner in the United States and Canada (or anywhere else). Don't tell them it's naturally fermented until after they're done eating it . . . see if anybody noticed!

- 3 cups fresh cranberries
- ½ cup chopped orange
- ¼ cup sugar
- 1 teaspoon sea salt
- ½ cup orange juice (freshly squeezed is best)
- ½ cup yogurt whey or water kefir
- Optional: dash of cinnamon, a little lemon juice

Place all ingredients in a food processor and "pulse" it until pieces are finely chopped, but not yet puréed. Transfer relish into a jar, stone crock, or bowl. Cover with cloth and let it sit for 2–3 days or until the taste is right for you (if you plan to serve it to fermentation newbies, then do not let it get too sour). If needed, add a little more sugar or honey to sweeten it up before eating.

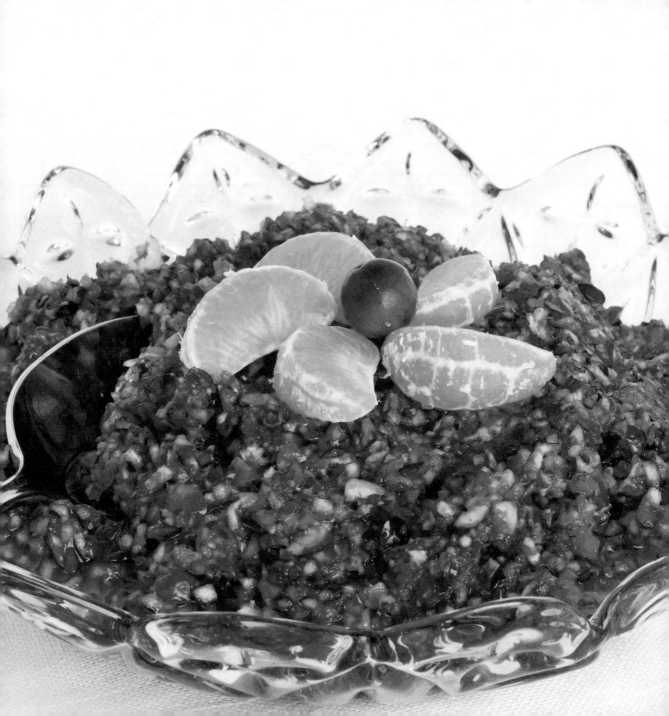

Greek Yogurt Cheesecake Bites (Gluten-free Option)

Makes one 8 x 8 inch cheesecake, 16 large bars, or 64 one-inch bites

This "no-bake" recipe replaces half of the cream cheese in cheesecake with Greek yogurt (homemade yogurt strained in tight cheesecloth for 3–5 hours or in a refrigerator overnight). The yogurt makes it more moist on top and less firm overall, so you need to be careful cutting it. For that reason, I recommend simply spooning the filling on top of the crust and then cutting it squarely into whatever serving size you want. This still is high in fat, sugar, and calories (hey, it's cheesecake!), but these evils are greatly reduced from regular cheesecake. Also, who needs a whole slice? See if a 1-inch bite gives you enough of a fix, and then invite 63 of your closest friends to share the rest.

Graham cracker crust:

- 2 cups graham cracker crumbles
- ⅓–½ cup melted butter
- ¼ cup sugar or substitute
- Pinch of sea salt

Press ingredients into bottom of an 8 x 8 inch pan. *Cooked:* Bake for 10 minutes at 400°F. *Raw:* Refrigerate for 1–2 hours.

Gluten-free crust:

- 1½ cups quick-cooking (instant) gluten-free oats, blended for 10 seconds on pulse
- ½ cup ground walnuts or pecans

- ½ cup brown sugar
- ⅓ cup to ½ cup melted butter
- Pinch of sea salt

Press ingredients into bottom of an 8 x 8 inch pan. *Cooked:* Bake for 10 minutes at 400°F. *Raw:* Refrigerate for 1–2 hours.

Filling:

- 1 cup (one 8-ounce/226-gram package) regular cream cheese, preferably a brand that contains live cultures, warmed to room temperature
- 1 cup Greek yogurt (homemade yogurt strained in tight cheesecloth for 3–5 hours or in a refrigerator overnight)
- ⅔ cup to 1 cup sugar or substitute
- ¼ cup lemon juice
- Zest of 1 lemon
- 1 teaspoon vanilla extract
- Pinch of sea salt

Prepare the crust in advance. Place all ingredients for the filling in a food processor or high-quality blender. Blend the filling until it is very smooth. Using a spoon or rubber/silicon spatula, scrape and pour filling mixture into crust. Smooth out the top, cover loosely (so cover does not stick to filling), and put cheesecake in the refrigerator to cool for 24 hours. If you have enough space in the freezer, you can put it in there for a few hours, too, for a firmer, semifrozen treat! Feel free to top the cake with fresh fruit, chocolate syrup, or any of the homemade soda syrups in this book (see soda chapter for recipes). Cut into bars or squares with a sharp knife and serve.

Chocolate Coconut Pudding

Makes about 3–4 cups

This pudding is made from puréed young coconut, which is cultured. You will need to use young green coconuts and not the hairy brown ones. In North America, young coconuts are often available in Asian and Latin American grocery stores; generally, their green skin has been hacked off, leaving them with a pointed or chiseled shape. Cut into the top with a heavy cleaver knife, pour out the coconut water and save it, and then scoop out the coconut meat. If you cannot find young coconuts, then you can use canned or frozen (and thawed) coconut purée.

- Meat of 3–4 young coconuts, scooped out (pour out the water and save this, too)
- 2 tablespoons yogurt whey or water kefir
- 1–3 tablespoons chocolate chips (melted and cooled slightly), chocolate syrup, or cocoa powder
- ½ cup or more coconut water
- Dash of cinnamon
- Optional: 1 tablespoon honey, maple syrup, or other sweetener

Purée all ingredients in a food processor or blender. Place pudding in a bowl or container, cover loosely, and let it ferment. Feel free to taste this and eat it whenever you wish, probably in around 2–4 days. With the rest of the coconut water, you can make a great probiotic drink by popping in some water kefir grains and culturing it into coconut water kefir.

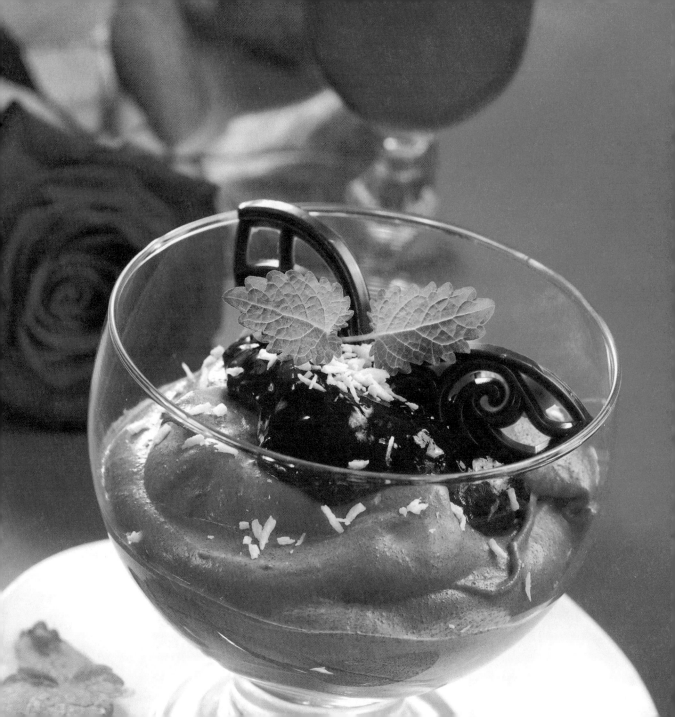

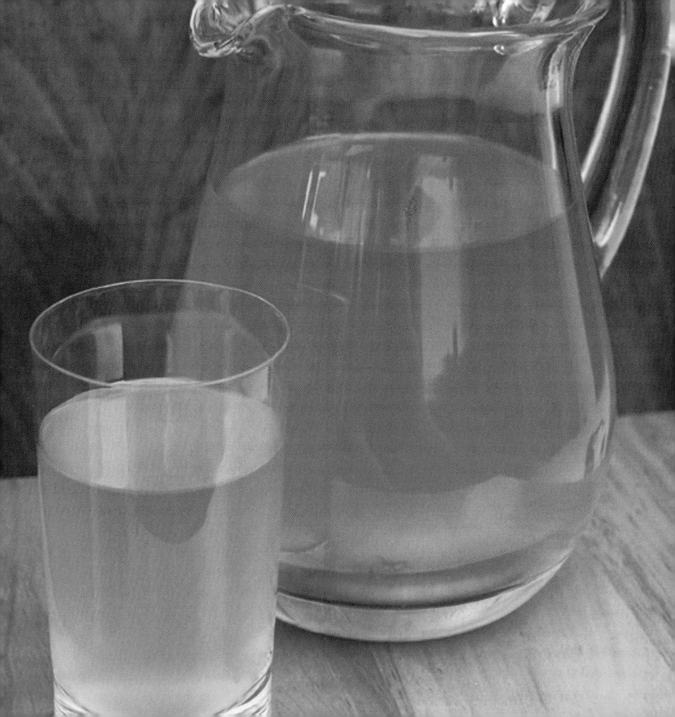

Chapter 13
Making Kombucha and Water Kefir (Tibicos)

Water kefir grains (tibicos) are merely kefir grains that have been developed to culture nondairy beverages. Rather than appearing white or creamy, tibicos are translucent. You can use them to culture sugar water, coconut water, or fruit juice into water kefir, coconut kefir, or cider. As far as their history and properties, they are identical to the kefir grains covered earlier. I include them here with kombucha, because they can be used in much the same way. However, tibicos can culture a drink in as quickly as 1–2 days, while the kombucha culture takes as long as 7–14 days.

Kombucha is a tasty drink made from culturing and fermenting sweet tea. It probably originated in Northeast Asia, specifically in the Manchurian region of China, but possibly in Japan. The first mention of kombucha appeared in Manchuria around 330 BC, while another story places it in Japan in 415 AD. However, because a seaweed tea in the region also carried a similar name, no one is sure that this referred to the fermented tea drink. Centuries later, kombucha emerged in a historical record in Russia, which may have been its actual place of birth.

The kombucha mother is a unique culture. First of all, it is the most visible of all SCOBYs, looking like a chunk of rubber or silicon. In addition, while kefir and ginger beer cultures mostly drop to the bottom of any liquid (at least until it gets carbonated), the much bulkier kombucha SCOBY floats on top of the drink. It can cover the entire surface area of the container and grow to an inch or more in thickness. The species of bacteria most responsible for the physical appearance of the kombucha mother is *Bacillus coagulans* (also known as *Lactobacillus sporogenes*). The porous, rubbery mat it creates provides a great living environment for up to a dozen additional kinds of yeasts and bacteria.

You can either obtain a kombucha SCOBY from someone who has some extra culture to share, order one online, or grow one yourself from a bottle of kombucha. Growing your own is fairly easy. Start with a store-bought bottle of kombucha, pouring this into a larger jar or plastic container along with some tea and sugar. After a few days, you will see a white film growing near the top of the liquid, which at first you might mistake for mold. Each day you check it, you will notice that the film has grown thicker, eventually becoming a deep mat that covers the top of your fermenting drink.

This flat blob is your very own kombucha mushroom, which you can use to ferment your own probiotic drinks and foods. Anytime you want to culture something new, you can gently move the mushroom to a new container. If it gets too big, you can cut it and divide the pieces. You can use your extra culture to ferment another drink, share it with a friend, or compost it. Used SCOBYs are great for your garden also, where beneficial microorganisms contribute to healthy soil, helping plants grow and stay healthy.

How to Make Water Kefir (Using Tibicos)

Water kefir is made by using tibicos (water kefir grains) to ferment sugar water. Most people use brown sugar, cane sugar, or maple syrup, or another wholesome

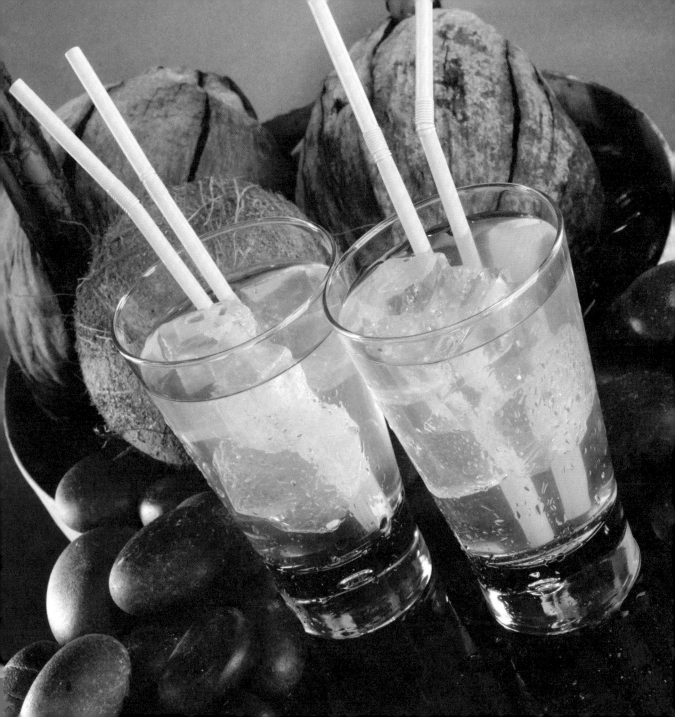

sweetener that provides more minerals than the depleted white sugar sold in stores. When the cultures do not have enough minerals available, they will not ferment effectively. Usually, water kefir grains (tibicos) are used to make water kefir, though milk kefir grains will work also.

Adding some sea salt (anywhere from a pinch to a teaspoon, depending on your preference) also can help ensure that minerals are present. Another option is to add some cut fruit or ginger to the ferment. This will supply a few more minerals as well as some flavor. But bear in mind that you will need to pick out the kefir grains later on from the fruit or ginger. And it is always possible to add flavor after the fermentation, once these grains are removed (see the chapter on making sodas for many postfermentation flavor possibilities).

As an alternative to sugar water, you can use coconut water from a young coconut, which contains enough sugar and minerals that it does not need any added sweeteners or minerals. Young coconuts and coconut water are increasingly popular. You can find both at many health food stores as well as Latin American and Asian food markets.

Water Kefir (or Coconut Water Kefir)

Makes 1 quart

Required materials:

- 1 large mixing bowl (glass, plastic, or wood, but not metal)
- 2 glass jars (quart-sized mason jars are good)
- 1 silicon spatula or wooden spoon

- 1 plastic strainer
- Cheesecloth, towel, or a sprouting lid for the jar

Ingredients:

- 1 quart of filtered (nonchlorinated) water or young coconut water
- ¼ cup (4 tablespoons) of water kefir grains (tibicos)
- Sweetener (not needed if using coconut water): ¼ cup of cane sugar, brown sugar, or maple syrup
- Optional: Chopped or sliced fruit of your choice or sliced ginger root
- Optional: Dash of sea salt

Process:

- Wash all equipment thoroughly before using.
- Place kefir grains in the jar, fill it with water, and gently stir in the sweetener.
- Optional: Throw in a dash of sea salt, which adds trace minerals to support the fermentation.
- Put the jar in an undisturbed place away from direct sunlight. Cover it loosely with the cheesecloth, towel, or a sprouting lid (which provides air circulation).
- Check your water kefir after 12 hours and again after 24 hours. Swish it around a little bit in the jar and then taste it with a clean spoon. If it's not sour enough for you yet, then give it another 12 hours. The fermentation will be faster in warm weather and slower when the air is cool. If you want to slow it down and fine tune your kefir, then you can put the whole jar in the refrigerator, where it will continue to ferment more slowly.
- Once you are ready to stop the fermentation, use the strainer over a bowl to strain out the kefir grains from the beverage. If you have also used fruit or ginger,

you must pick out the kefir grains from these; my favorite tool for this is wooden/bamboo chopsticks. Your kefir can be enjoyed immediately or stored in a jar or plastic container in the refrigerator.

- Reuse your kefir grains immediately in a new batch of sugar water or else store them for up to two weeks in the refrigerator (sitting in some sugar water).

How to Make Kombucha

To make kombucha, you simply mix up some sweet tea, put it in a jar, place your SCOBY in it, and cover it with a loose lid or a towel for aeration. Kombucha SCOBYs float near the top. For a quart of kombucha, use 2–4 tea bags and about 1/2 cup of white sugar, which should be cooled to room temperature before you add the SCOBY. Yes, in the other chapters I recommend more wholesome sugars, but for kombucha, white sugar balances nicely with the tea.

Kombucha SCOBYs do not ferment as fast as kefir grains, so it probably will take from 1–4 weeks to brew a batch. The length of time varies based on the temperature, the SCOBY's potency, and your taste preference. As with other fermented beverages, you can drink it early at a slightly sweeter stage or you can let it ferment for a longer period for a stronger taste.

It's good to put your brew in a relatively warm place, where the air temperature is 65–82°F. Anything much colder than that may cause the yeast to shut down and go into hibernation. I find that the top of my refrigerator stays a bit warmer than room temperature. In colder weather, you can use a heating mat of the type used to grow seedlings.

Checking for Proper Fermentation

Your nose and the little bubbles should tell you if your kombucha is fermenting properly. But if you suspect something has gone wrong and the culture has failed, then you need to check it more closely. The best method of investigation is to use pH test strips. If, after 3–4 days of fermentation, the pH of your fluid is not in the 2.5–3.0 range, then it is not acidic enough and something has gone wrong. Dump it out, sterilize everything, and start again with a new culture. Also, if there is a strong kerosene smell coming from the kombucha, as opposed to a yeast or vinegar smell, that means something else has gotten in there and you need to dump it.

Fizzy Kombucha

If your kombucha is not as effervescent as you would like, you can conduct a secondary fermentation in a bottle. To fuel this second stage, you can use juice (which provides a nice flavor), or else use some more sweet tea. Either way, you will end up with a kombucha soda.

Take a plastic bottle with a tight-fitting lid, such as a soda or water bottle. (You can use a glass jar or bottle also, but it is easiest to check the air pressure in a plastic vessel.) Fill it three-quarters of the way with your fermented kombucha and top this off with some additional juice. Tighten the lid and leave this at room temperature to continue fermenting. It probably will be ready in 2–7 days, but check it every day or so.

If you used a plastic bottle, then checking it is as simple as squeezing the sides of the bottle. If it has really puffed out so that squeezing is difficult, your drink should be ready. Open with caution, since the contents may be under pressure. Unless you've shaken the bottle, it really should not explode on you, but there will be a release of air pressure as there is when opening any soda bottle. Taste and decide if it's fizzy enough for you. If not, tighten the lid and give it another 12 hours or so.

Storing and Reusing Your Kombucha SCOBY

Storing a kombucha SCOBY is easier than storing kefir grains, simply because it takes longer to ferment a batch. This means that you can start fermenting some sweet tea with a kombucha SCOBY and just leave it for as long as a couple of weeks. The fermented liquid may be too acidic to drink, but your culture should still be alive after that time and you can begin using it again. While you can store your SCOBY in the refrigerator, this can cause the yeasts to go dormant, so the above method is better.

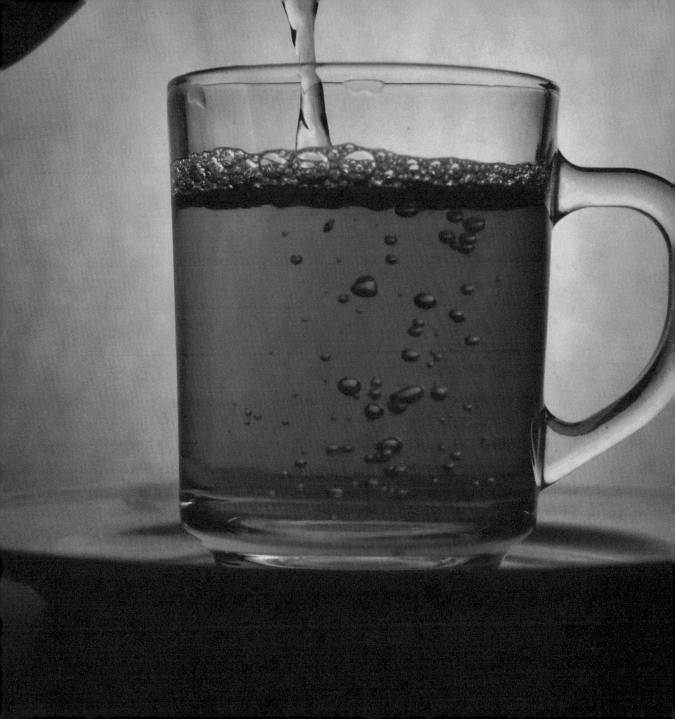

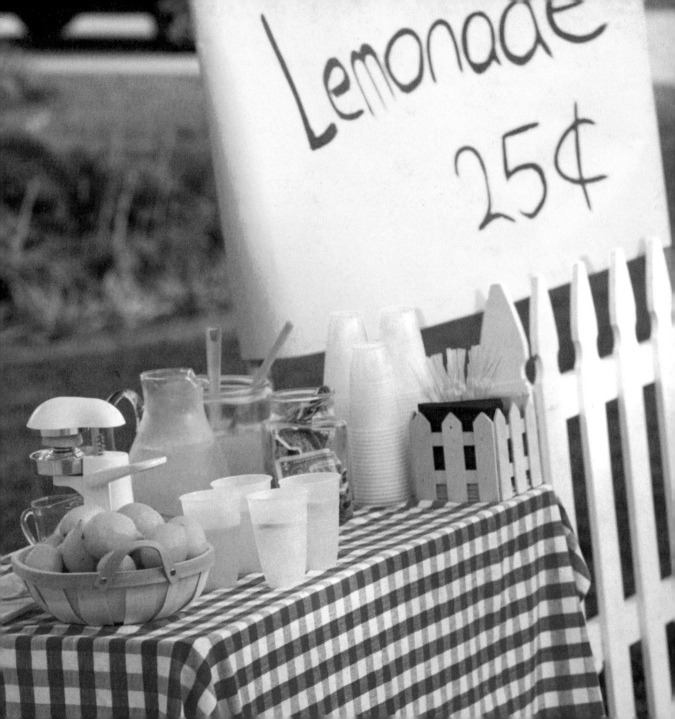

Chapter 14
Probiotic Lemonade, Watermelon Kombucha Cooler, and Pineapple Tapache

This section is reserved for three special drinks. They could be considered sodas or smoothies, but all three are made a bit differently from the other drinks. We'll just call them the author's favorites!

Probiotic Lemonade

Makes about 2 quarts

This only takes a few more minutes than dissolving one of those chemical-filled lemonade envelopes in water. This drink is probiotic from the start by virtue of the cultured drink (kombucha, cider, etc.) you have added. But if you can wait for a richer ferment, prepare the drink in advance and let all the ingredients stand together for 24–48 hours. Also, see the separate Lemon-Lime Soda recipe, which is similar. Try this lemonade on your kids!

- Juice of 5 lemons
- ½ cup kombucha, cider, water kefir, or yogurt whey
- 1½–2 quarts water
- ¼–½ cup sugar or honey

Mix together all ingredients and let the drink sit in a jar or container for 24–48 hours or until it reaches desired sourness. If it's too sour, feel free to thin it out with more water or add extra honey or sugar. Garnish with a sprig of mint or slices of lemon.

Watermelon Kombucha Cooler

Makes about 2 cups

- 1 cup ripe watermelon
- 1½ cups kombucha or water kefir
- Honey or sugar, to taste

Blend watermelon to purée it. If chunks remain, strain them out. For a frozen drink, freeze watermelon or purée first, then blend with kombucha or water kefir. If you do not freeze the purée, then you can stir it directly into the kombucha.

Pineapple Tapache

Makes 3–4 quarts

This delicious beverage from Mexico may well be my favorite drink in this book. The recipe involves fermenting a whole pineapple (cut into chunks) in sweetened water with spices. You can culture it with water kefir grains (tibicos), yogurt whey, or cider. Otherwise, just let the naturally present bacteria culture it themselves. Traditionally, people cut up the peel and put this in to get plenty of bacteria. If

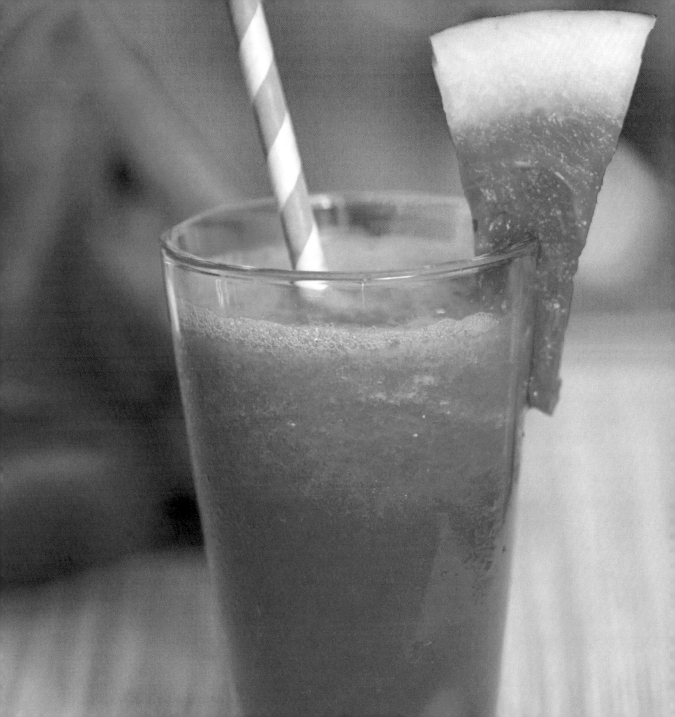

you use the rind, then please cut off the bottom and discard this part, as ripe pineapples often have a little mold at the base of the core.

- 3–4 quarts water
- 1 fresh pineapple, peeled and cut into chunks
- 3 cups natural cane sugar or brown sugar
- 1 teaspoon vanilla extract
- 1 cinnamon stick or one teaspoon ground cinnamon
- Optional: 1 tablespoon apple pie spice

Put the pineapple chunks in a very large container or jar, covering it with water. Use enough water to cover the pineapple—probably about half (2 quarts) of your water. Also add the sugar and spices. Then add your kefir/yogurt/cider culture, if you use any. Cover loosely and let it ferment. After 48 hours, add another quart of water and cover it loosely again. Let it sit for 12 hours this time before tasting. If it is sour enough for you, then drink some and refrigerate the rest. If it needs more time, add more water and give it an additional 12 hours to ferment. It should be ready at that point, and if it is too sour, you can add a little sugar, honey, or apple juice. You can eat the pineapple chunks or compost them. I feed some to my backyard chickens (the subject of another book) who love pineapple. They need their probiotics, too!

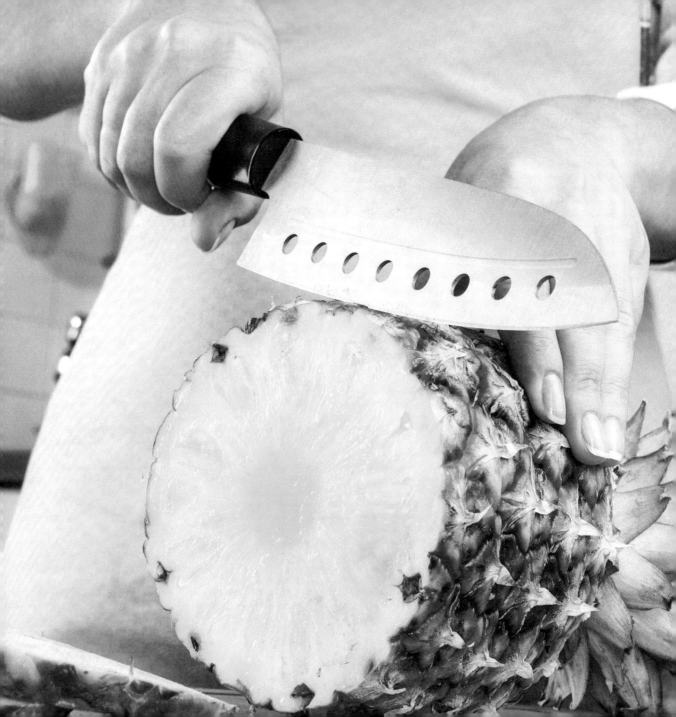

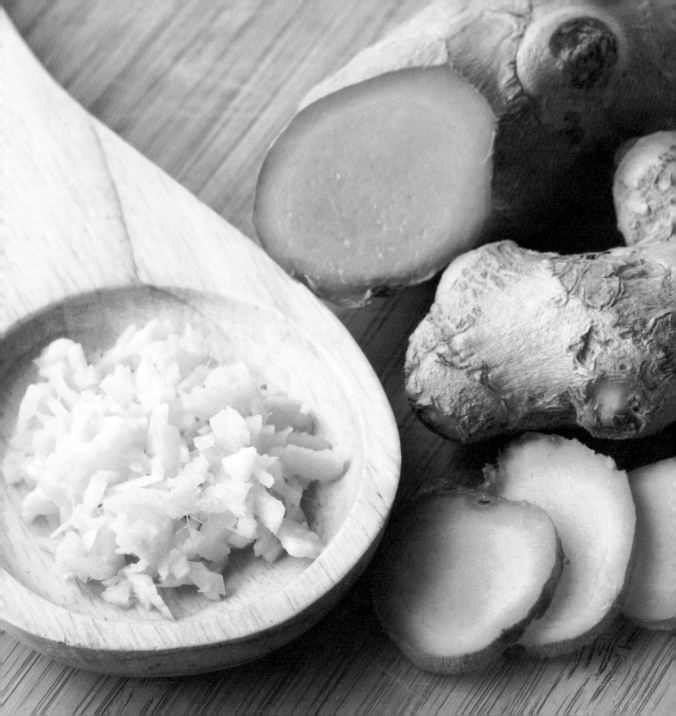

Chapter 15
Ginger Beer and Rejuvelac

Like kefir and kombucha, real ginger beer is cultured by a unique SCOBY with its own fascinating story. The ginger beer culture, also known as the ginger beer plant, once fueled a large brewing industry in Britain and several of its colonies. Today, after nearly going extinct, the ginger beer plant is available again. This chapter covers ginger beer made with this authentic culture. Also, there is a recipe for rejuvelac at the end of this chapter; it is a fermented grain drink that is useful mainly as a base culture for other drinks and foods.

As with kefir grains and kombucha mushrooms, the ginger beer plant can culture just about anything. Most people use it to make a (mostly) nonalcoholic ginger beer. There is an imitation version out there called a ginger bug, but the ginger bug generally involves just growing some wild yeasts. I'm sure they ferment things just fine, but they are not the authentic ginger beer plant culture. Authentic ginger beer has a very low alcohol content, probably below 1 percent.

Separately, this book covers "ginger ale" in the chapter on making natural sodas. For the sake of simplicity, I have given the name ginger ale to our ginger-flavored natural soda (with a base of water kefir, kombucha, or rejuvelac). The name "ginger beer" means the beverage that is fermented directly by the authentic ginger beer plant culture. In the real world, these two names are used rather interchangeably, and these two drinks might come out tasting pretty similar, but I think the ginger beer plant deserves its own drink.

No one is quite sure where the ginger beer plant originated. There are claims that it came from India or Africa before being brought to the Caribbean. In the 18th century, it became popular in Jamaica, and British breweries began making boatloads of it. Significant quantities were exported to the United States, Canada, Australia, and elsewhere in the British sphere of influence. Soon, these countries began to brew their own; call it ginger beer independence.

Toward the end of the 19th century, as brewing yeasts became better understood and more widely available, the drinks probably became more alcoholic and less probiotic. The ginger beer plant then faded into obscurity and virtually disappeared. It was discovered decades later in Germany, where a few determined souls continued to keep it alive. Today, there are amateur fermenters around the world who have ginger beer plants. You can obtain one through a local group or online, though these SCOBYs are nowhere near as prevalent as kefir grains or kombucha mushrooms.

The old stoneware bottles for ginger beer remain collectors' items in many places. I have one from a Syracuse, New York, brewery that made "English brewed" ginger beer. This particular brewery began in England in the late 19th century and expanded to the United States in 1900. It was closed in 1920 with Prohibition, so the brew probably included its fair share of alcohol by then. Most likely, the brewery was using brewing yeasts, which were capable of making ginger beers with alcohol contents of up to 11 percent. The real ginger beer plant is capable of creating a little more alcohol than some other SCOBY cultures (perhaps around 1–2 percent, probably since there is no aceto acid bacteria when fermentation starts), but an isolated yeast is far better for making an alcoholic drink.

The ginger beer plant is a rather unusual SCOBY culture. While kefir grains and kombucha mushrooms often contain ten or more species of yeast, lactobacteria, and aceto acid bacteria (a mix that can vary), the ginger beer plant contains just two organisms. It is a symbiotic community made up of a yeast called *Saccharomyces florentinus* and a bacterium called *Lactobacillus hilgardii*. Nothing more.

How the ginger beer plant ended up with just two organisms in its mix is a mystery, but it may have developed from kefir grains, which often contain the same two species in the ginger beer plant. Ginger beer plants are more difficult to obtain than either kefir grains or kombucha mushrooms, but they are available. If you cannot find one locally, check online. In the appendix of this book, you will find some good resources, including a list of website sources for live cultures. At the time I wrote this book, two of them sold ginger beer plant.

Ginger Beer (Authentic)

- Ginger beer plant
- 1 quart water
- 1–2 inches ginger, peeled and finely chopped
- ¾ cup to 1 cup sugar

Combine all ingredients in a large jar or container. Cover loosely and let ferment at room temperature. Check it after 24 hours, and move it to the refrigerator when ready, but it may take 2–3 days to ferment to your liking. When it's ready to cover and move to the refrigerator, then strain out the ginger beer plant and put this in your next batch of ginger beer. It is a fairly sensitive culture, so I do not recommend trying to store the it in the refrigerator; just save at least a small amount of it and keep a continuous culture going.

Rejuvelac

Rejuvelac is a fermented beverage made from sprouted cereal grains, such as wheat, barley, rye, oats, triticale, millet, amaranth, quinoa, brown rice, wild rice, or buckwheat. People have been making fermented drinks with grains for thousands of years, but the raw food advocate Ann Wigmore is credited with popularizing rejuvelac as part of a holistic health diet. It's pretty sour and definitely qualifies as an acquired taste unless you add some sugar, honey, or other sweetener. Alternatively, this makes a great base ingredient for sodas, or you can mix it with juice, and it can be used to culture anything else in this book.

- ½ cup organic grains such as wheat, rye, barley, or oats (whole-seeded, not ground or cracked)
- Water
- Optional: 1 tablespoon yogurt whey or water kefir

Rinse the grains. Put them in the jar or container and cover them with water. Let them soak overnight. In the morning, drain the water from the grains, rinse them, and put them back in the jar. The rinsing prevents mold. Continue to rinse twice per day for 1–2 days, until grains form small white tails, indicating that they have sprouted. Rinse them once more and put grains in the large container. You could use the same jar if it's big enough (be sure to rinse before reusing).

Cover the grains with one quart of water. Add yogurt whey or other culture, if you choose to use this (if not, the natural yeasts and bacteria on grains will ferment the water). Cover the container loosely, checking it by tasting every 24 hours. This fermentation normally takes 1–3 days, and the later you let it go, the more sour it will be. Then pour out the liquid, which is the consumable part. The grains have left the better part of their nutrition in the liquid and are spent, so you can compost them. Feel free to add some sweetener or combine the rejuvelac with juice to make it drinkable.

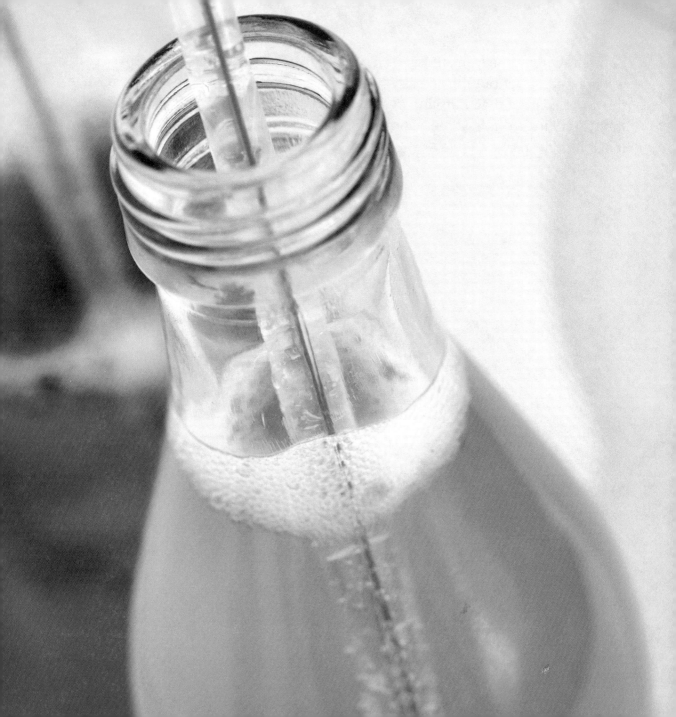

Chapter 16
Homemade Sodas and Fruit Ciders

*P*lease be mindful that cultured soda and cider becomes naturally carbonated. If you place it in a bottle, jar, or other container with a lid, then the contents can be under high pressure, which will increase with additional fermentation. In extreme cases, bottles can explode. And drinks certainly can burst out the top of these vessels when opened. Check your soda fermentation often, do not shake contents, and use plastic bottles if you are worried about breaking glass. Please be careful and stay safe!

Most of us like fizzy drinks. Root beer, cola, ginger ale, and sparkling apple cider: what do these drinks have in common? All are sweet, sparkling beverages. And traditionally, all of them were brewed with probiotic cultures that provide a natural source of effervescent bubbles. When you make them at home, these drinks retain far more goodness than your average soda pop. Imagine being able to call your soda pop a health food!

Yes, this is an alternate universe with no high fructose corn syrup or pumped in CO_2 bubbles. Here, we enjoy sodas and ciders that are low in sugar, rich in protein and B vitamins, teeming with rich probiotics and enzymes, and naturally sparkling as a result of fermentation. Plus, you can add whatever flavors and healthful herbs you want, making a custom soda to suit your tastes. If you've never tried cultured cranberry cider, almond sarsaparilla, or lavender lemon soda, you're in for a treat. This chapter will cover a few basic recipes, and from there, you can create your own.

You can brew ciders and sodas using any of the cultures we have covered. Kefir grains, a kombucha SCOBY, a ginger beer plant, or even yogurt whey will get the job done.

My first choice of a culture for soda or cider is water kefir grains (tibicos). Water kefir grains, which are adapted to culturing sugary water, will work quickest and have the best chance of maintaining a stable culture over time (assuming you plan to keep these grains after your first ferment). These grains can ferment a beverage in as little as 1–2 days, while a kombucha SCOBY will take up to 1–2 weeks.

Natural Ciders (Probiotic, Fermented Juices)

Making ciders is extremely simple. Begin with a bottle of your favorite juice (apple, grape, berry, etc.). Just open the bottle of juice and pour some into a jar for the fermentation. Then add your culture, which could be a kombucha SCOBY or a tablespoon or two of kefir grains, ginger beer plant, or yogurt whey. Then cover the bottle or jar loosely with the lid or cover it with a towel or cheesecloth, holding the latter in place with a rubber band. Leave the cultured juice out of direct light where it can remain still for a few days.

Depending on the temperature and the strength of the culture you used, your cider can ferment in just a day or two (though a kombucha culture will take longer). Remain on the lookout for little air bubbles forming and feel free to taste a bit whenever you want to test it. Near the beginning, it will be sweet from the sugars in the juice, and as it ferments, the sweetness will turn sour from the conversion of sugars to acids. When you like the taste, go ahead and drink it, saving the rest in

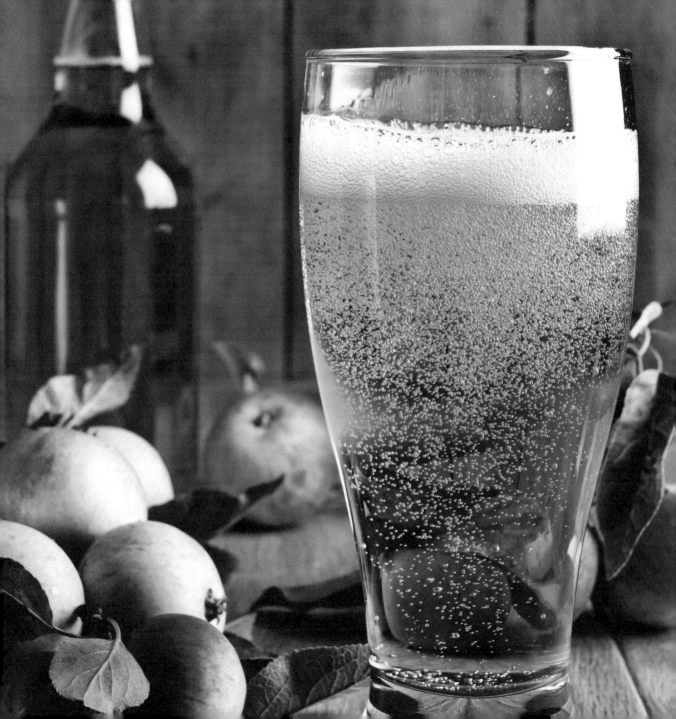

the refrigerator to enjoy over the next few days. Here is a quick explanation of the different levels of flavor/body and how to achieve them:

Sweet and Mild

The juice begins with a sweet and mild flavor, so if you want to culture this lightly and get very little fermented taste, then simply drink it within the first day or two.

Mildly Fermented

To achieve this taste, let it go a little longer. This may be 2–3 days with kefir grains and a bit longer with other cultures. Taste it once a day until it has the fermented flavor you like, but still a bit of sweetness.

Strongly Fermented

Let it go an extra day or two for the most concentrated probiotic benefits. This is the strong, sour taste of a heavily fermented beverage, and it will start to get quite yeasty as these organisms begin to dominate. Your cider will have a bit of alcohol (probably under 1 percent) and should have the effervescence of a little natural carbonation.

Sweet and Sour

It's cider, not medicine! To get the full probiotic benefits of complete fermentation, plus the sweetness that makes it enjoyable, just take out a few ounces of juice at the beginning and save this in the refrigerator. Ferment the remainder, and once this is nice and sour, strain out any kefir grains or SCOBY, and then mix in the reserved juice. Alternatively, you can add a pinch of sugar or a spoonful of honey, maple syrup, or molasses at the end. Voila, sweet and sour, the best of both worlds!

Fizzy Bottling

If your cider is not fizzy enough, try bottling it for a secondary fermentation like we do with the sodas. Take a plastic bottle with a tight-fitting lid, such as a soda or water bottle. (You can use a glass jar or bottle also, but it is easiest to check the air pressure in a plastic vessel.) Fill it halfway with the fermented cider and top this off with some additional juice. Tighten the lid and leave this at room temperature to continue fermenting. It probably will be ready in 24 hours, but check it within 12 hours. If you used a plastic bottle, then checking it is as simple as squeezing the sides of the bottle. If it has really puffed out so that squeezing is difficult, it is probably ready. Open with caution; you could have a bomb in your hands! Unless you've shaken the bottle, it really should not explode on you, but there will be a release of air pressure as there is when opening any soda bottle. Taste and decide if it's fizzy enough for you. If not, tighten the lid and give it another 12 hours or so.

Pumpkin Jack-O-Cider

Makes varying quantities (depending on size of pumpkin)

Making cider in a pumpkin? What a cool idea! Here is a great way to use an extra pumpkin, enjoying its terrific flavors and nutrition. I recommend using the tibicos or yogurt whey as cultures, since you need to make this ferment quickly and beat the mold by a couple of days. The cider is delicious. Sorry, you cannot carve a face on this one or put a candle inside! Well, maybe after you drink it . . .

- 1 pumpkin
- Enough apple juice to nearly fill the pumpkin
- 2 tablespoons kefir grains or yogurt whey
- Optional: Cinnamon stick, 1-inch piece of peeled ginger, or dash of pumpkin pie spice mix

First, use a large knife to cut the top off a pumpkin. Then remove the seeds with a large spoon, just like you do when making a jack-o-lantern. Once the seeds are out, use the spoon to gently scrape the inside edge, loosening a little of the pumpkin meat and leaving this at the bottom. Next, fill the pumpkin nearly to the top with apple juice and add some tibicos grains or yogurt whey as a culture, plus optional spices, and put the top back on loosely. Within 2-3 days, you will have a very unique, flavorful, and healthy cider. Please make sure you remove the cider and drink or bottle it before the pumpkin starts to mold, since the mold may begin in less than a week.

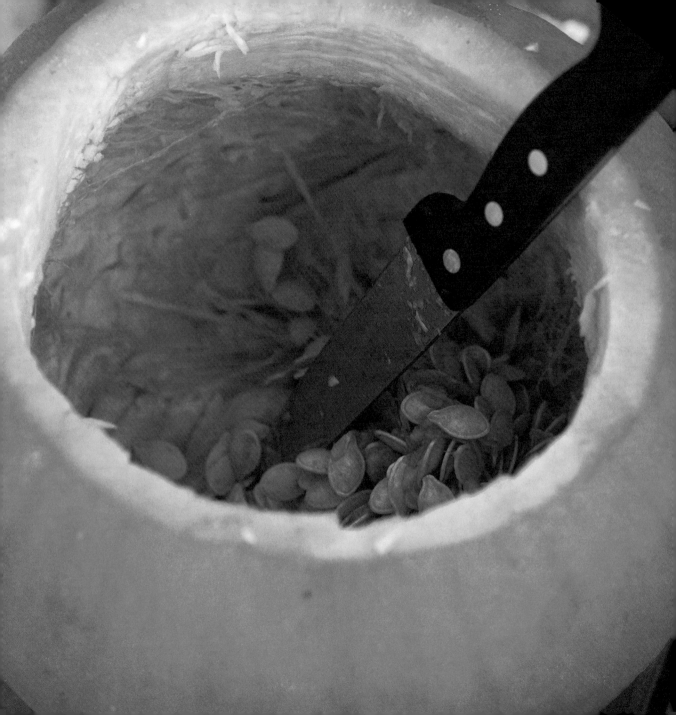

Saving Your Cider Culture

When you pour off the juice, you can do so with a strainer to catch any kefir grains, ginger beer plant, or SCOBY. A kombucha SCOBY often floats in the liquid, so another way to catch it is to grab it with tongs. These solid cultures can be saved for the next fermentation project. Yogurt whey or dried cultures will dissolve in the juice, so you can just drink it all or save a few ounces to mix with the next batch.

Air Locks Are Very Useful

Home brewing supply stores sell a cheap device called an air lock (sometimes known as a water lock or pressure lock). This is a plastic valve with a rubber gasket that fits over the mouth of a bottle. There are some different styles (three-piece, S-shape, and bubble locks), but they work the same way. You mount the device on the bottle that contains your brew, often with the help of a rubber bottle stopper (bung) that has a hole to fit the lock, then you fill this lock with a small amount of water or other fluid. Some people use a sterile alcohol like vodka. The liquid stays in the lock, enabling CO_2 to escape as the drink ferments, while preventing any outside air, dust, mold spores, or insects from getting into the brew.

Air locks are optional. A loose-fitting lid will work fine also. But air locks make your job easier and help prevent any contamination. At the time of writing this book, a set of three air locks is about the same price as a sandwich. I usually buy mine on Amazon, but you can also find these locks at some health food stores as well as any home brewing supply store.

Homemade Sodas

Home brewed sodas are really a treat. They are much, much healthier than any high fructose, artificially flavored, chemically preserved, and unnaturally carbonated soda on the market. Plus, making your own soda gives you the freedom to add any flavor you like. If you like root beer, cherry cola, ginger ale, cream soda, sarsaparilla, or lemon-lime, you can make it at home. You can also make lavender, pumpkin pie, mandarin orange, molasses, and a whole lot of other soda flavors that are not available in stores.

There are three steps to making your own natural soda. First, you will brew up the fermented base, which can be either kombucha, water kefir, rejuvelac, or ginger beer. Alternatively, you can just use brewer's yeast or baker's yeast. Of course, these single culture yeasts do not have the probiotic benefits of the traditional cultures described in this book.

Second, you will add some flavoring to this fermented base. Juices, fruit syrups, and herbal extracts are good flavoring candidates. Below the soda recipe that follows, you will find a list of flavoring sources, which include fruit syrups and juices, extracts of herbs and spices, and ready-made natural flavoring extracts such as cherry cola or cream soda flavoring. Third, you have the option to conduct a secondary ferment to add some carbonation and finish off the bottling of your soda. Here is the process.

Naturally Cultured Soda

(Recipes for soda syrups follow this recipe)

This recipe makes slightly more than one quart. In addition to the materials and ingredients needed to make water kefir, kombucha, rejuvelac, or ginger beer (which are explained in the chapters covering each of these drinks), you also will need some plastic bottles or jars with tight-fitting lids. Soda or water bottles with screw top lids work well. It is easier to check the inside pressure of plastic bottles by squeezing them, but you could use glass bottles or Mason jars and just take a small risk that they might burst. If you use extracts for flavoring and still want to do a secondary ferment, then you should also have some extra plain-tasting fruit juice (such as apple juice), fruit syrup, or maple syrup ready to add to each bottle.

Ingredients:

- 1 quart of fermented base, such as water kefir, kombucha, rejuvelac, or ginger beer
- ½ cup soda syrup (or other syrup flavoring, per its label directions)
- Extra juice, maple syrup, or fruit syrup, to taste

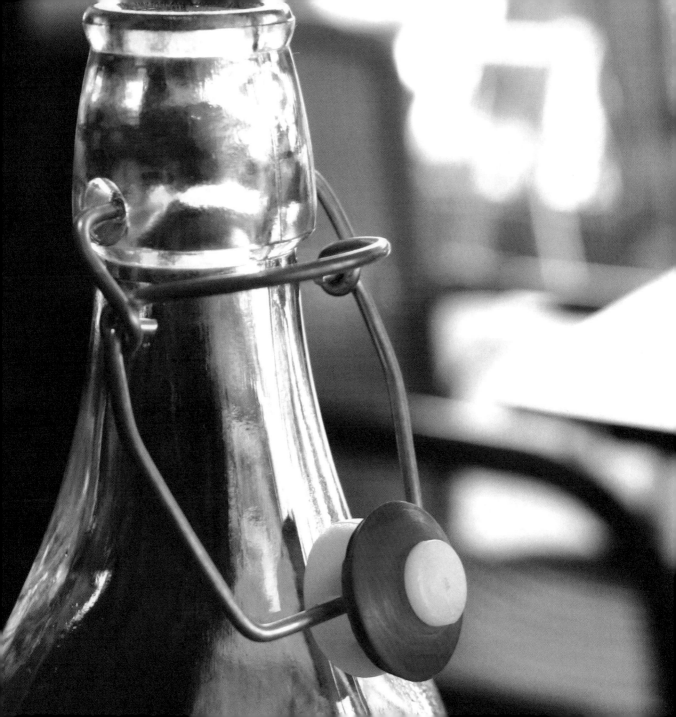

Process:

- Make a batch of water kefir, ginger beer, kombucha, or rejuvelac as your fermented base for the soda. Please refer to the directions in the separate chapters on each of these. Bear in mind that kombucha will be the slowest among them, while the others are all pretty fast cultures.
- Once you have made the base (following the directions in the appropriate chapter), pour it into each of the bottles or jars. Leave enough room for the fruit juice/syrup and any flavoring you wish to add.
- Put the lids on tightly. You can leave the soda bottles out and check them every few hours or put them in the refrigerator, where they will keep fermenting more slowly. Kombucha soda should be left out.
- Check your sodas by squeezing the sides of the plastic bottles. Once they are firm with the expanded pressure from the ferment, open them and taste. If you use glass bottles or jars, you will need to open them to check the fermentation. Beware of the pressure inside, which will release when you open the bottle. Once you taste the soda, only you will know when it is ready. If should be nicely fermented and effervescently carbonated, yet still sweet enough for you. If it's not strong enough, put the lid back on and let it ferment a few more hours. If it's too sour, add a little more of your juice or syrup.
- Drink it and enjoy! Even the kids should love it!

Soda Flavoring Sources

Fruit Syrup: Any fruit or berry can be made into a fruit syrup, which combines with the fermented base to make a great soda. Soft fruits such as berries, grapes, peaches, apricots, cherries, plums, figs, and mangoes make particularly good syrups. Fresh fruit is best, but you can rehydrate dried fruit to make an effective syrup as well.

Take about two pounds of your favorite fruit, wash it, and chop it (except for berries and small fruit, which do not need to be chopped). Remove the pits from any stone fruit (like peaches, plums, cherries, and apricots) you use. Do not worry about the seeds in grapes or berries, since the syrup will be strained later. If the fruit you use is purely sweet and does not have any tartness to it, you can add some lemon or lime juice to balance this if you wish.

Put the fruit in a pan, adding 1 cup of water and 1 cup of sugar. Cook the fruit on medium-high heat, stirring it regularly and adding more water as needed to prevent sticking and burning. After 15–20 minutes, the mixture should look like a soupy jam. If any chunks remain, try to mash them in.

Let the fruit mixture cool, then strain it into a bowl or container. This is your fruit syrup, which can flavor any soda. If you have a lot of it, you can store it in a bottle or jar in the refrigerator for a few days. For longer storage, put it in the freezer in a freezer-safe container. You can also follow a standard canning procedure used for jam, preserving the syrup in jars for whenever you need it.

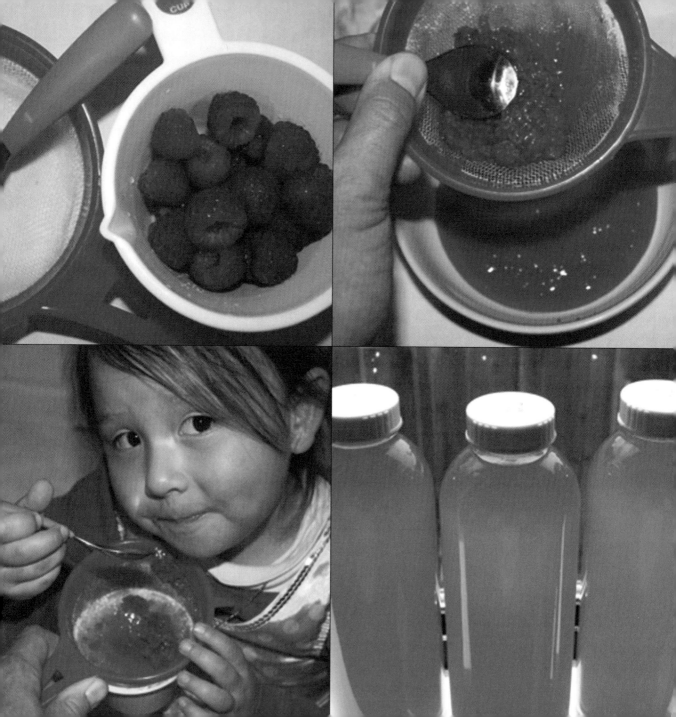

Ginger Syrup for Ginger Ale: You probably will not need as much of this to get the flavor you want. Nevertheless, to make a great ginger ale, follow the directions above for making a fruit syrup, using fresh ginger root instead. Peel it, chop it, and boil it with some water and sugar to make a strong, tasty, healthful soda flavoring.

Fruit Juices: Juices can be used to flavor sodas as well. Grape, apple, and cranberry juices are good bets, and you can experiment with any others you like. In general, the more intense flavors are best. For example, dark purple grape juice has a great flavor, while some of the transparent, filtered apple juices just taste like sugar and water. Then again, there are really good apple juices that have full flavor as well.

Extracts of Herbs and Spices: Mint, lavender, and chamomile are three kinds of herbs that make nice flavor additions in any soda. Then there are spices such as cinnamon, cloves, allspice, and curry, which might make interesting additions to a beverage. Please see the last section of this book for Lavender Soda and Pineapple Tapache recipes.

There are several different ways to get herbs and spices into your drinks. You can put a cinnamon stick in for a couple of minutes. You can boil fresh or dried herbs like mint or lavender into any fruit syrup, or skip the fruit and just boil the herbs in sugar water to make herb syrup. Another option is to use herb tea bags of mint and chamomile for an herbal infusion. If you steep them in boiling water for a while, the tea water can be used to make syrup or simply added to the soda with as much sweetener as you want.

Ready-Made Flavoring Extracts: You probably have vanilla extract in your cupboard already. Next to the vanilla in supermarkets you can usually find almond, peppermint, and coconut extracts. Since homemade sodas (combining fizzy water with syrups) have become popular in recent years, there are more soda extracts available than ever before. Check online merchants (like those mentioned in the appendix) if you cannot find what you want locally.

Here are recipes for several delicious soda syrups.

Making Soda Syrups and Soda Pop

To make soda syrup, combine all ingredients, stir well, taste, and adjust sweetness as needed. Many of the herbal syrups need to be cooked first in order to extract the flavors, while some fruit syrups can be made raw. Once finished, you can use the syrup immediately or store in the refrigerator in a container.

To make soda pop, add ¼ cup to ½ cup soda syrup to 2 cups of kombucha or water kefir. Then place this mixed base + syrup in a bottle, jar, or container with a very tight-fitting lid. Leave a little room on top. Cover and let it ferment at room temperature or in the refrigerator. Check room temperature soda every few hours, tasting until your soda has the right level of carbonation or effervescence. Refrigerated soda may take 1–3 days to reach the right stage, but it can happen in less than one day also, so check it regularly.

If it tastes too sour by this point, then add a little more soda syrup, maple syrup, or sugar to the top of each bottle/jar/container before consuming.

Lemon–Lime Syrup

This gives your soda an intense citrus flavor. If you prefer a sweeter or milder soda, then increase the sugar or use less syrup. Use any ratio of lemons to limes, or even just one kind of fruit, if you prefer.

- 1–2 lemons, juice and zest
- 4 limes, juice and zest
- 1 cup water
- 1 cup sugar

Combine all ingredients. Use it raw.

Cherry Almond Syrup

- 2 cups cherries, fresh or frozen
- 1 cup water
- Sugar (½ cup for sour cherries, ¼ cup for sweet cherries)
- 2 teaspoons almond extract

This one you need to boil for 15 minutes, blend or mash the cherries, and strain. If you prefer to keep the cherries raw, then freeze them first, thaw, blend, and strain the purée. Also for a raw version, boil a little of the water and stir in the almond extract; then let the water cool. That way, any alcohol is removed that might interfere with the culture.

Concord Grape Syrup

Make your own fresh juice from some flavorful grapes (such as Concords) or buy a bottle of grape juice.

- 2 cups grape juice
- 1 tablespoon lemon zest
- ½ cup sugar (or less if grape juice is very sweet)

Combine all ingredients. Use it raw.

Maple Cinnamon Syrup

- 2 cups maple syrup
- 2 cinnamon sticks

Boil maple syrup in a small pan. Add cinnamon sticks while syrup is hot. Let it sit for 1 hour.

Mint Syrup

- 1 cup mint leaves
- ½ cup sugar
- 1½ cups water

Cook on medium heat, turn off heat, and then let it sit for 1 hour.

Licorice Syrup

- 2 cups water
- ¼ cup dried licorice root, chopped
- ½ cup sugar

Cook on medium heat for 15 minutes, turn off heat, and then let it sit for 1 hour.

Raspberry Rhubarb Syrup

- 2½ cups raspberries
- 2 large rhubarb stalks, chopped
- 2 cups water
- 1–2 cups sugar

Bring water to a boil, add rhubarb, then simmer on medium heat for 15 minutes. Add raspberries and simmer for 15 minutes more, then cool and strain.

Chai Spiced Syrup

- 2 cups water
- ¼-inch piece of fresh ginger
- 1 cinnamon stick
- 2 cardamom pods
- 2 whole cloves
- Optional: ⅛ teaspoon black peppercorns

Bring to boil and simmer for 15 minutes. Cool, strain out spices, and serve.

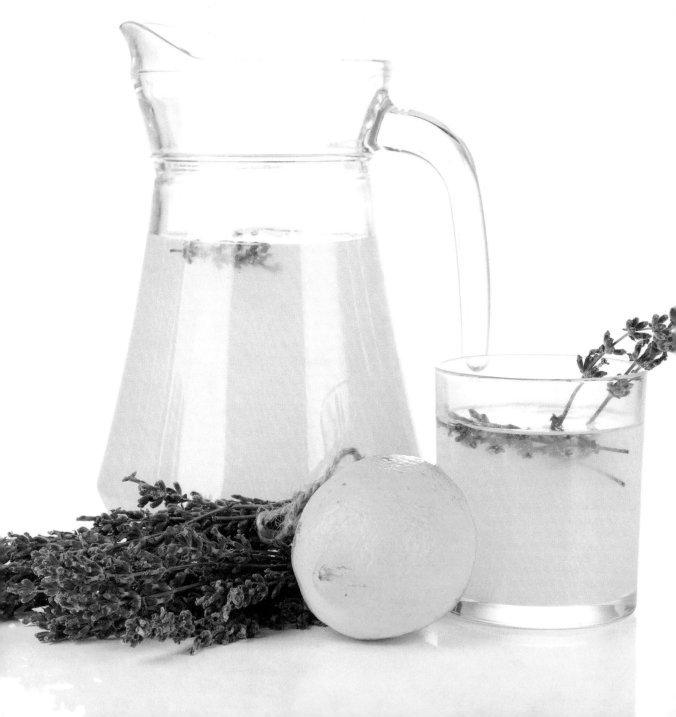

Lavender Syrup

- 1 cup water
- ½ cup sugar
- ¼ cup dried lavender

Bring to a boil, simmer on medium heat for 15 minutes, then cool and strain out lavender.

Cola Syrup

This is adapted from a recipe by chef Lorraine Elliott, author of *Not Quite Nigella*. It is a simplified version of the very complex formulas of well-known commercial colas. And this one tastes a little more natural! I substituted lemon juice for the citric acid, but since lemons vary in acidity, you may want to taste this and adjust the lemon juice to fit your taste preference. Don't forget that your soda base (kombucha or water kefir) will be sour also, so if the syrup ends up on the sweet and mild side, that might be fine.

- 2 cups water
- 2 cups brown sugar
- 2 tablespoons maple syrup
- Zest of 1 lemon, 1 lime, and 1 large orange (very finely grated)
- 2 teaspoons coriander seeds, crushed in mortar and pestle
- 1½ teaspoons dried lavender
- 4 sections of a whole star anise

- 1 vanilla pod, split
- 1 cinnamon stick
- 1 teaspoon fresh ginger, finely minced
- 2–3 teaspoons lemon juice

Place all ingredients in a medium-sized pot. Simmer for 20 minutes. Cool and strain out the herbs.

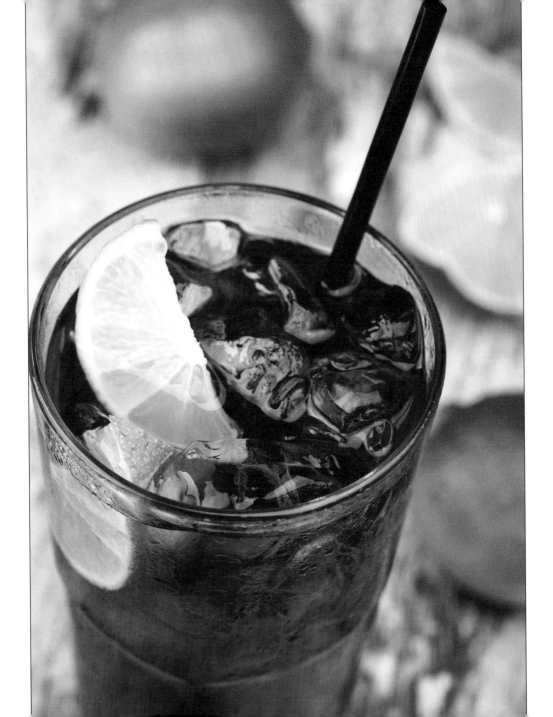

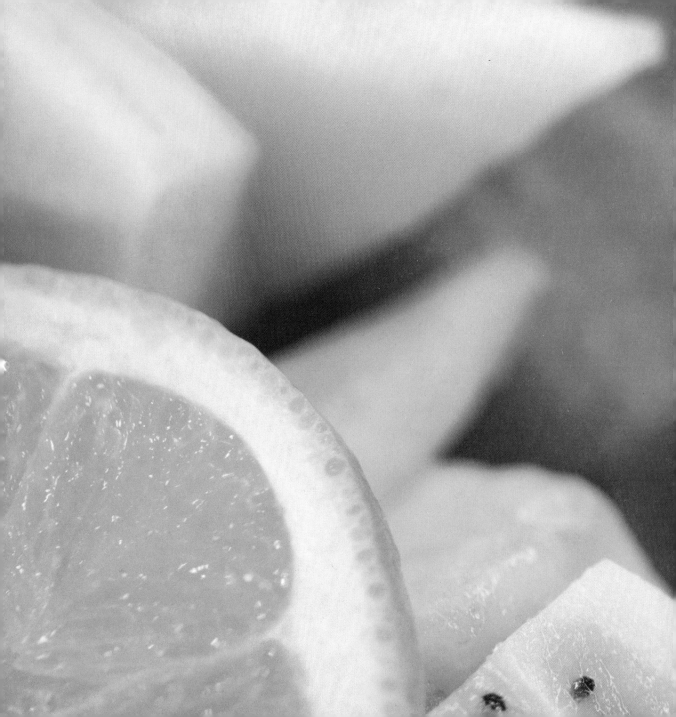

Chapter 17
Smoothies, Parfaits, Frozen Drinks, and Yogurts

Smoothies are just plain delicious. These drinks provide an enjoyable way to get both your nutrients and your probiotics. You can use yogurt, kefir, water kefir, kombucha, rejuvelac, or cider as a probiotic base for smoothies, blending this base with your favorite fruit for a tasty beverage. Smoothies are a great probiotic option for anyone who does not like the taste of other fermented foods. If you have kids and are looking for a great way to slip them something healthy (such as green juice powder, vegetable juice, or vitamin powder), then try disguising it in a probiotic drink that everyone will love!

This section also includes recipes for a parfait, frozen yogurt, and a frozen drink. In fact, you can make a parfait or a slushy frozen drink from nearly any one of the smoothie recipes. Just go easy on the liquid ingredients and aim to make the blended ingredients into more of a purée than a liquid. Most people eat parfaits with a spoon rather than drinking them. Pour the blended purée into a parfait glass, tumbler, wine glass, or whatever vessel you want to use, and then sprinkle on any "topping" ingredients you wish to add, such as granola, chopped nuts, shredded coconut, or dried fruit.

If you would like different layers in your parfait, then wash the blender between uses and simply make some different short-on-liquid smoothies. This book's parfait recipe lists several different fruits that help create a rainbow of colors. And of course, you can blend some chocolate syrup, chocolate chips, or cocoa powder for a choco layer, peanut butter for a peanut layer, garlic for a . . . okay, I'll stop there. Alternate with dry topping ingredients to create additional layers.

To make a frozen drink, you can freeze the fruit that is called for in the smoothie recipe. Alternatively, you can add a handful or two of ice. Some people blend up all the other ingredients first and then add the ice last, pulsing it in the blender until the ice or frozen fruit is small enough for you. The best blenders can make a good frozen drink, but it is difficult to get them quite as slushy as the commercial blenders. There even is one "instant" frozen yogurt recipe that is just as simple as a smoothie: it uses frozen fruit to get the ice crystals, so there is no waiting time at all between making and eating.

If you have made your own smoothies before, then you know how simple smoothie making can be. You may even have your own recipes already, which can be modified easily to incorporate more probiotics. If you have never made a smoothie before, then you can start with one of my recipes in this chapter. From there, please feel free to make modifications based on your own preferences and what local fruit you have available. Experiment a little and you may improve on my recipes, creating your own smoothie masterpieces.

To make a smoothie, all you need is a blender, some fruit (fresh or frozen), some probiotic yogurt or fermented drink, possibly some fruit or veggie juice, and any other ingredients you wish to add. Additional ingredients can include leafy green vegetables, green juice powder, protein powder, nuts, frozen yogurt, honey, jam, or ice. Hey, you can even throw in some garlic and anchovies if you want—it's your drink!

The word *smoothie* was part of my vocabulary at an early age. When I was a kid, my parents used to make one with bananas and milk. Once I was old enough to operate a blender, I started making my own smoothies, usually with a few more ingredients. I rarely use recipes to make smoothies, and rarely make the exact same smoothie twice. This is not because I am some culinary genius; it's just that smoothies are very forgiving. You can make them a different way each time and still come out all right. There is plenty of room for error, and room for experimentation.

Each of the recipes in this chapter provides a starting point for smoothie making. The proportions of ingredients are the most important aspect, but even these can vary. Some people like a thick smoothie that goes down like a glass of milk, while others prefer a thick concoction you can stand a spoon in. My recipes will produce drinks that are a bit on the thick side, but generally drinkable through a straw (assuming you have a good blender that can reduce the fruit to tiny chunks).

Once you have the basic proportions figured out, then feel free to substitute ingredients and innovate. For example, if you see a recipe for a pineapple smoothie, when your local plums are in season, then go ahead and use plums instead. Fresh, ripe, seasonal, local fruit is always best.

If the fruit you use is quite different from the one in the recipe, then you can make adjustments. For example, pineapple has more fiber and is drier than a juicy, ripe plum. Pineapple is also quite acidic, while most plums probably are sweeter than all but the ripest pineapples. So if you use plums, you could cut down on any other sweet ingredient the recipe calls for (such as honey or apple juice) and you might not need as much liquid. However, if your plums are purely sweet without much background flavor, your smoothie may end up tasting rather insipid (sweet, but lacking in flavor). Plums are one of my favorite fruits, but most of them do not make a good smoothie on their own. Consider adding extra yogurt or kefir, a little orange or cranberry juice, or even a twist of lemon or lime to create more of a tangy taste.

Frozen fruit works just as well in smoothies and frozen desserts as fresh fruit. If you want a cold smoothie or instant frozen yogurt, frozen fruit is perfect. I sometimes freeze fresh fruit just so I can put it in smoothies. Besides, good quality fruit is scarce in the winter and early spring. My family drinks fewer smoothies during the cooler months than at any other time of the year, simply because good fruit is harder to get or more expensive at these times. A smoothie is a great way to enjoy good fruit that was frozen in its prime.

Frozen raw fruit still contains most of its nutritional goodness (including enzymes) as well as the same fresh fruit flavor. During the summer, when the cherry, blueberry, strawberry, blackberry, and peach crops peak, we either pick our own or buy boxes of the best quality fruit at a discount. Then we wash, trim/pit, chop, and freeze these fruits in double zipper bags or freezer containers. I have tried this with other fruits as well, but these ones are the winners with our kids.

Here is my rundown on various fruits and what they add to a smoothie or frozen dessert.

Apples are one of my favorite fruits, but they do not blend very well. You may be comfortable cooking them first (think of apple butter), while I prefer my ingredients raw. Raw apples create a smoothie with crunchy texture, which may make them a better fit for a parfait or frozen yogurt. Another option is to juice them first, because apple juice is a terrific sweetening ingredient in smoothies and blended foods.

Bananas provide an unbeatable thick texture as well as a great background sweetness. Though I am not what you would call a banana person (I rarely eat them), I think they are nearly essential to a good smoothie. Fortunately, they are available in most regions at most times of the year. Put a banana or two in your smoothie and it's hard to go wrong.

Blueberries, Cranberries, Blackberries, and Raspberries can add terrific flavor and healthy antioxidants to smoothies. There is nothing like that wild blackberry taste, and in many places, you can harvest bucket loads of blackberries for free in the countryside. High quality, ripe raspberries can make a great smoothie addition also. However, both raspberries and blackberries are very seedy, and if the fruit is not of premium quality, then they will add a mostly sour taste without much aroma. I will only use these at their peak of flavor and ripeness. If you find these berries make too seedy of a smoothie, then feel free to strain out the seeds. As far as blueberries and cranberries go, it is hard to go wrong with using them in smoothies. They are also very easy to freeze during their peak season, which allows you to use blueberries or cranberries year-round at times when they are expensive or absent from stores. Cranberries, of course, are pretty sour, so use them in moderation and add some sweetener.

Cherries add a beautiful color, a good range of nutrients, and plenty of antioxidants to smoothies. I have a guillotine-style fruit stoner, and even with that contraption it becomes a pain in the neck to pit all those cherries. But when winter comes, the pitting is worth every minute, because we can enjoy ripe cherries year-round in smoothies and frozen desserts. We wait until the peak of the season when they are on sale, buy several pounds' worth of dark, ripe cherries at a discount, then wash, pit, and freeze them. If you use sour cherries, you will need extra sweetener, such as honey.

Dates are a great sweetening option in smoothies. Though they are very high in antioxidants, you can only use a few dates in a smoothie because of the amount of sugar. Dried dates blend fairly well unless they are really dried out.

Figs are really seedy. I love eating them, but I don't put them in smoothies. Well, maybe one or two really ripe ones!

Grapes, in general, are rather disappointing in smoothies, though some people like them in a chunky frozen yogurt. Aromatic grapes like Concords can make a great juice that tastes fabulous in smoothies. But as far as blending them in? The skins get in the way, as do any seeds. I suggest just using the juice if you want a grape flavor, unless you do not mind eating or straining out bits of skin and possibly seeds. Of course, if you have some seedless, thin-skinned table grapes around and want to throw in a handful or two, they make a nice sweet addition to any blended confection.

Guavas are good in smoothies as well, adding a terrific flavor and a slightly grainy pear texture (unless you just use the juice). They require varying amounts of sweetener, since some guavas are quite sweet on their own, while others are almost as sour as lemons.

Kiwis should not be combined with dairy because they contain a powerful enzyme that creates a bitter taste. If you make a smoothie based on yogurt or kefir, then leave out the kiwis, but they are good in a vegan smoothie that is milk-free or uses an alternative such as almond or soy milk. Ripe kiwis have it all: sweetness, tartness, and a wonderful smoothie texture after being puréed in a blender.

Lemons and Limes are slightly less useful than their sweeter citrus cousins. You can use a little lemon or lime juice in a smoothie, but only a little before it gets quite sour. I particularly love the taste of limes and Meyer lemons, so I often use them to provide a tangy, flavorful twist. But if you use much more than a few drops, then you are making one sour smoothie (unless you add some sugary ingredient and go the lemonade route). Fermented base ingredients, like yogurt, already are pretty sour. By the way, use some zest from the peel in any food or drink if you want to incorporate the taste or lemons and limes without the sourness.

Mangoes are one of the best possible fruits to add to a smoothie. They have a great flavor and plenty of sweetness. Best of all, puréed mango makes a custardy texture that thickens up a smoothie. This is one of the few fruits that can both replace a banana and flavor a smoothie all by itself. Mangoes are related to poison ivy and many people (including me) have an allergic reaction to them. If you cut off the skin and the few millimeters or so on the outside of the fruit's flesh (those closest to the peel), then this removes most of the offending substance. I can tolerate mangoes in small doses and my body seems to tolerate them when they are combined with a thick yogurt or kefir; most other people can enjoy them in larger quantities. One other plus with mangoes is that sometimes the grocery stores in the United States (and probably elsewhere) have a good crop of them for sale in the springtime when local temperate fruits are not ready yet. Mangoes provide a welcome source of fresh fruit flavor and are a very dense source of nutrition.

Melons are mostly water. Even the sweetest and most flavorful are turned to juice in a blender. This is fine if you treat melons as juice. Like pears, most melons will not thicken your smoothie very much, unless they are less than ripe (in which case they add crunchy chunks). The recipe for instant frozen yogurt recommends using melons, and it actually tastes great when they still are a little bit chunky.

Oranges, Grapefruits, and Mandarins/Tangerines provide an important acidic tang to smoothies as well as some sweetness. Oftentimes, I taste a smoothie that I've just blended and conclude that it's missing something. After squeezing in a ¼ cup or so of fresh orange juice, I taste it again and decide it is perfect. If you like the taste of grapefruit, as I do, then feel free to use as much fresh grapefruit juice as you like. I use mandarins and tangerines just like oranges for their juice. The bonus with mandarins and tangerines is their terrific flavor and aroma.

Peaches/Plums/Nectarines/Apricots/Hybrid Stone Fruits can be great in smoothies, especially when they are at their peak of ripeness, sweetness, and aroma. At less than their peak, they can add more tartness than flavor, so even if you compensate by sweetening things up with some honey or apple juice, your smoothie can be a little on the acidic side. Also, make sure they are fully ripe so that they actually purée, unless you do not mind chunks.

Pears are sweet additions to smoothies when fully ripe. Grainy pears will add a slightly earthy texture to your smoothie, while the creamiest ones seem to disappear into juice. Even the ripest and softest pears, though, will not create body the way that a banana does. Think of pears as more juicy ingredients, and of course they need to be fully ripe to purée well. Asian pears have a texture more like apples, which makes them more difficult to blend well than the soft European and American varieties.

Pineapples and Papayas are two tropical fruits that taste great in smoothies. Like kiwis, both have powerful enzymes that can begin curdling milk right away. So again, I would go with a nonmilk smoothie, though yogurt seems okay. Both of these fruits are delicious in smoothies, papayas having a custardy texture and pineapples being a bit more fibrous (but quite blendable).

Strawberries are an excellent smoothie fruit. Fully ripe strawberries make a very fine purée, which not only flavors but thickens a smoothie. In my area, we have access to fresh strawberries for much of the year, and they are quite cheap at their peak. As a result, we either have fresh or frozen berries year-round, and they end up as either a starring or supporting ingredient in nearly every smoothie we make. Strawberries are not as seedy as raspberries and blackberries, but you can strain out the seeds with a fine mesh strainer if you want.

With other fruits I have not covered, from mangosteens to cherimoyas to pawpaws to sapotes to currants to gooseberries, I just don't have a lot of experience with these in my area. Feel free to experiment!

Strawberry Banana Shake

Makes 5–6 cups

Where I live in Northern California, we can get fresh, local strawberries several times per year. The rest of the time, we keep frozen berries for use in smoothies. And of course, bananas always seem to be available in stores. So this is our classic smoothie recipe. Often, we vary it by adding or substituting other fruit that is in season or in the freezer. Use two bananas if you like it thicker and sweeter. Since strawberries can vary in sweetness/sourness, feel free to adjust the honey or sugar as needed.

- 1 cup milk or CRASH alternative
- 1 cup yogurt
- 3 cups ripe strawberries
- 1–2 large, ripe bananas
- ¼ cup orange juice or apple juice
- Honey or sugar to taste

Place all ingredients in a blender. Blend, taste, adjust with additional honey or sugar, and serve.

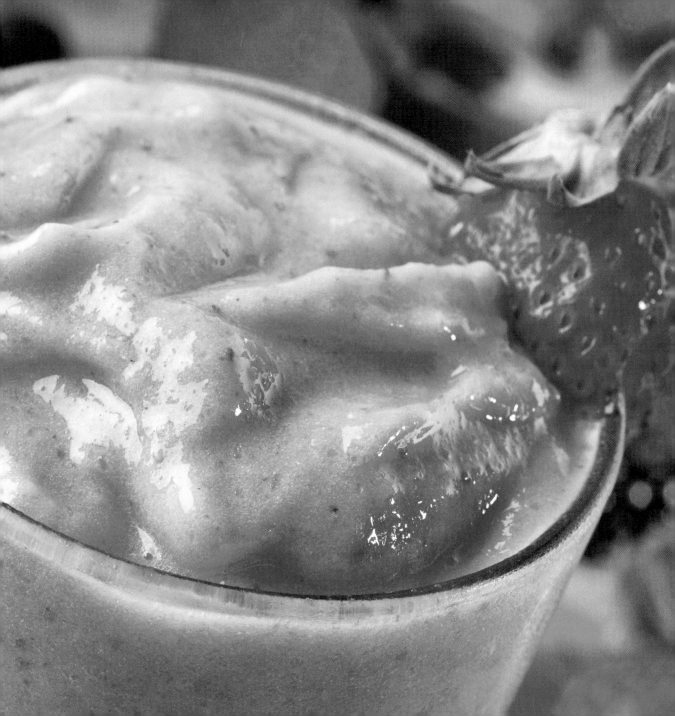

Mango Lassi

Makes 3–4 cups

If you like mangoes, this drink is a tropical dream. If you have ever had a mango lassi at an Indian restaurant, this is a close homemade rendition. Many restaurant versions use canned mango juice, which has an intense sweet taste and added sugar. Of course, you can buy a can of this at an Asian grocery store and use it instead of mangoes. But using ripe mangoes will create a fresher taste with plenty of sweetness (and I mean really ripe ones, since anything less is sour and remains chunky after blending). This recipe tastes great with coconut milk as well—it's kind of a mango-colada!

- ½ cup yogurt or cottage cheese
- ¾ cup milk or CRASH alternative
- 2 large ripe mangoes, peeled and cut
- Optional: 1 teaspoon honey (or more if your mangoes are a bit sour)
- Optional: Dash of ground cardamom or nutmeg

Place all ingredients in a blender. Blend, taste, adjust with additional honey or sugar, and serve.

Blackberry Smoothie

Makes 4–6 cups

This smoothie, with its vibrant purple-blue color, is my pick for the most beautiful drink in this book. It also tastes great, particularly if you use ripe berries. You can

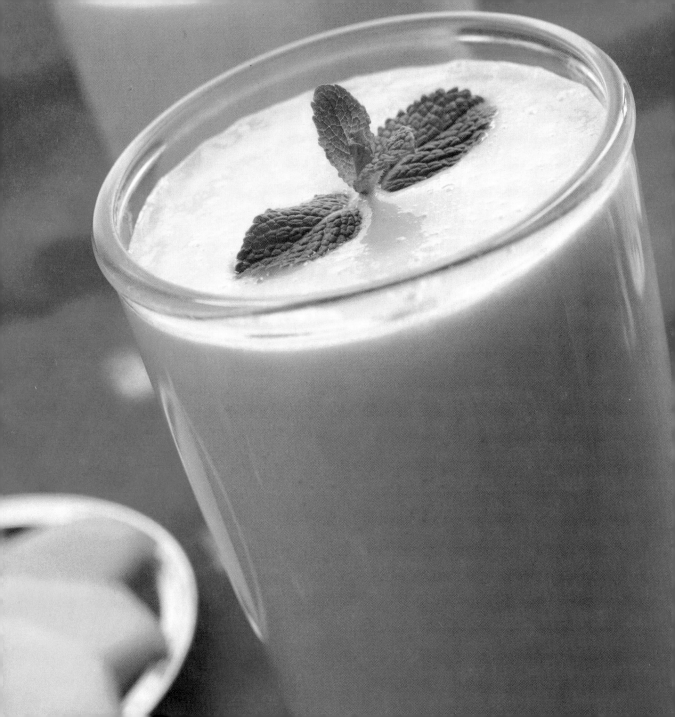

use blueberries or raspberries if you prefer. There are a lot of seeds, so if you don't like this aspect, then run it through a strainer after blending.

- 2 cups blackberries
- 1 cup yogurt or kefir
- 1 banana
- 1 cup cider or apple juice
- 2–4 tablespoons honey (less if you use apple juice)

Place all ingredients in a blender. Blend, taste, adjust with additional honey or sugar, and serve.

Cherry Kombucha Smoothie

Makes 3–4 cups

Feel free to substitute blueberries, blackberries, or raspberries for the cherries. Adding yogurt makes this tarter, while a banana sweetens it. Use a little honey or sugar if your fruit is too tart.

- 1 cup kombucha
- ½ cup yogurt and/or 1 ripe banana
- 1½ cups frozen, pitted sweet cherries

Place all ingredients in a blender. Blend, taste, adjust with additional honey or sugar, and serve.

Peanut Butter and Jelly Smoothie

Makes about 4 cups

If you love eating a PB&J sandwich, try drinking one! You can use almond butter, cashew butter, or a nut-flax butter for this if you prefer. Raw foodies can use raw nut butter. Whatever your favorite nut butter, I recommend creamy and unsalted (if you can find it) versus the chunky and salted varieties.

- 2 ripe bananas
- ½ cup blackberries, blueberries, or pitted cherries
- ½ cup milk or CRASH alternative
- ½ cup yogurt or kefir
- ¼–½ cup peanut butter

Place all ingredients in a blender. Blend, taste, adjust with additional honey or sugar, and serve.

Pina Colada

Makes 3–4 cups

- 1 cup coconut milk or coconut kefir
- 1 cup yogurt or cottage cheese
- ½ teaspoon coconut extract
- 2 cups pineapple, chopped, fresh or frozen
- Optional: Honey or sugar to taste (particularly if pineapple is sour)

Place all ingredients in a blender. Blend, taste, adjust with additional honey or sugar, and serve.

Krautberry Smoothie

Makes about 4 cups

Here's one for kraut diehards. The addition of sauerkraut gives this smoothie a tangy, salty kick. Omit the banana if you prefer a savory smoothie. Add your favorite cliché here: This will put hair on your chest . . . it will separate the men/women from the boys/girls . . . it's an acquired taste . . . you won't know what you're missing unless you try it.

- ¼–½ cup sauerkraut
- 1 banana
- 1 cup yogurt or kefir
- 1 cup strawberries, blackberries, raspberries, or blueberries (or use other fruit, fresh or frozen)
- 1 cup apple juice, cider, kombucha, or water kefir

Place all ingredients in a blender. Blend, taste, adjust with additional honey or sugar, and serve.

Mint Mojito Smoothie

Makes 3–4 cups

Ah, the refreshing Cuban-Caribbean combination of mint and fresh lime. If you find it a bit too sour, go easy on the lime juice.

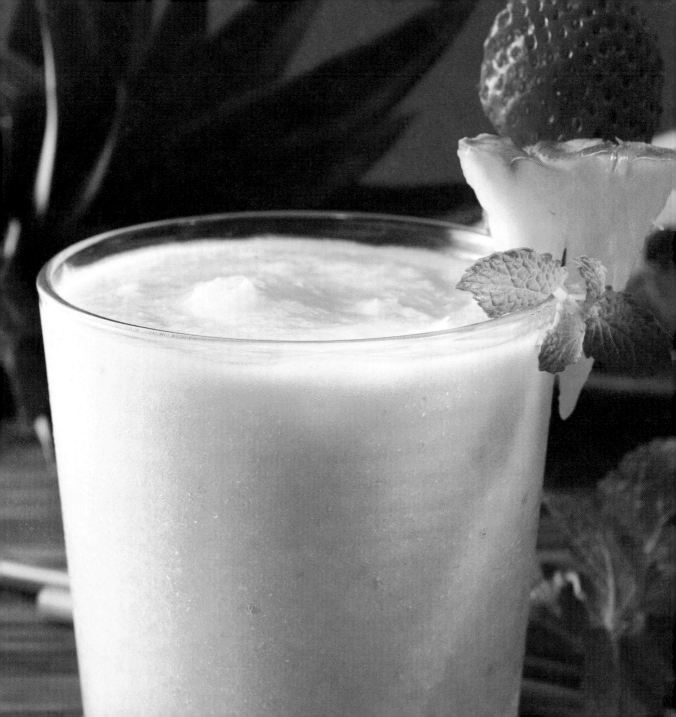

- 1 cup kombucha, water kefir, or rejuvelac
- 15–20 leaves of fresh mint, removed from stems
- 1 cup yogurt
- 1 banana
- 1 avocado, peeled and pitted
- 2 tablespoons lime juice
- Optional: Additional lime juice if you like it really sour. To add additional lime flavor without the acidic kick, you can add the zest of 1 lime instead.

Place all ingredients in a blender. Blend, taste, adjust with additional honey or sugar, and serve.

Red, White, and Blue (or Rainbow) Fruit Parfait

Makes about 4–5 cups

Try this healthy and festive-looking dish for a holiday or anytime. The parfait is layered with different colored fruit purées, most of them blended with honey-vanilla yogurt. So the only challenge is washing your blender in between colors. This recipe goes for the red, white, and blue look, but you can use other colors for a rainbow effect: orange from mangoes or peaches, yellow from pineapple, green from kiwis, and purple from dark plums, blackberries, or cherries. Just remember (in case you did not know) that kiwis, papayas, and pineapples have very powerful enzymes of their own that can curdle dairy products and make them bitter, so if you use these fruits, a layer of 100 percent fruit purée (no yogurt) may be best. Use frozen fruit for a more refreshing treat or fresh fruit for a healthy breakfast treat. To make this more of a meal, feel free to add additional layers with solid ingredients, such as granola, nuts, or your favorite breakfast cereal.

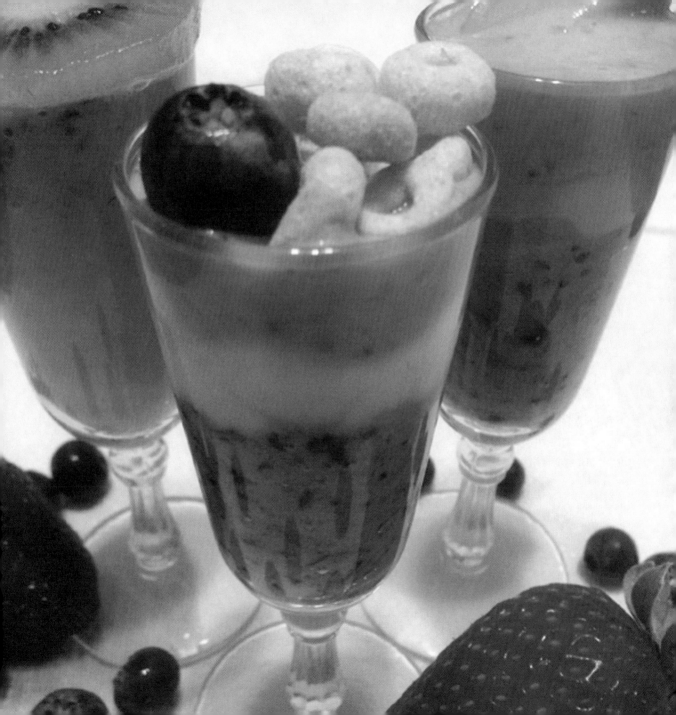

White layer and base:

- 3 cups yogurt
- 2 tablespoons honey
- ¼ teaspoon vanilla extract

Blend all ingredients. Then remove 2 cups of the yogurt mixture and reserve this. Use the remaining yogurt mixture in the blender to make your blue layer.

Blue layer:

- 1 cup blueberries
- 1 cup yogurt mixture (see above)

Add blueberries to the rest of the yogurt mixture that remains in the blender. Blend thoroughly. Remove blue mixture and set aside. Wash out blender.

Red layer:

- 1 cup strawberries *or* ½ cup strawberries + ½ cup watermelon
- 1 teaspoon honey or sugar (if the berries are sour)
- 1 cup yogurt mixture

Blend thoroughly. Then assemble parfait in a tall glass, wine glass, tumbler, or parfait glass. First, spoon or pour blue layer into bottom third of glass. Sprinkle any solid topping (such as granola) over this if you wish. Then cover it with the white layer, up to two-thirds of the height of the glass. Again, sprinkle in any solid layer you wish to add. Top with the red layer and garnish with extra berries.

Frozen Chocolate Mocha Latte

Makes about 5–6 cups

To make this recipe, you will need a good blender that can really crush the ice. Or else you can convert it to an iced coffee by just adding the ice cubes after you blend up the rest of the drink (it will be more intense this way, so feel free to dilute it with additional water or milk). Begin by making some strong coffee. You can use a coffee maker or brew it by hand. Use 2½ cups water and at least ½ cup of ground coffee to brew some strong stuff. Any variety of coffee works. Optionally, you can add some sliced almonds or almond butter for an almond mocha flavor (with or without the chocolate ingredients).

- 2½ cups strong coffee, freshly brewed
- 1 cup yogurt
- 1 cup ice cubes
- ¼ cup whipped cream (or substitute milk for lower-fat version)
- 1 tablespoon chocolate syrup
- 1 teaspoon chocolate chips
- ¼ teaspoon vanilla extract
- Sugar or honey to taste
- Optional: 1 tablespoon almond butter or sliced almonds, plus replace the vanilla with almond extract

Put all ingredients (except ice) in a blender and blend them on a high setting until puréed. Taste to see whether additional sugar or honey is needed. Then add ice and blend on a pulse setting until the ice has reached your desired size.

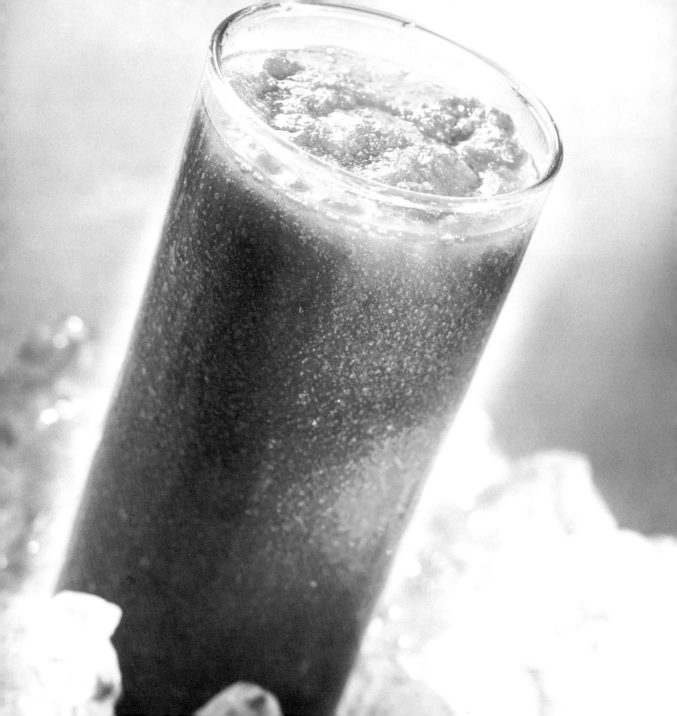

Some people like a crushed ice drink with fairly large ice cubes in it that are semi-incorporated, while others prefer to get the ice crystals as small as possible without them dissolving. Few home blenders are capable of rendering the slushy ice drinks that commercial blenders can create, but this will be close to the real thing!

Please see additional smoothie recipes in the next chapter, where they are classified as green drinks.

Blueberry Frozen Yogurt

Mmmm, it's good. Makes about 6 cups.

- 3 cups blueberries
- 2 cups yogurt
- ½ cup sugar
- 1 cup milk
- 1 tablespoon lemon juice

In a saucepan, bring berries, lemon juice, and sugar to a boil, then turn to medium heat and simmer for 10 minutes, adding a little water if needed to keep the mixture from drying out. Combine yogurt and milk in a blender or food processor, add berries, and mix (on a quick-pulse setting if you want to maintain any chunkiness). Then follow directions in the Peach Ice Cream (page 131) recipe for freezing.

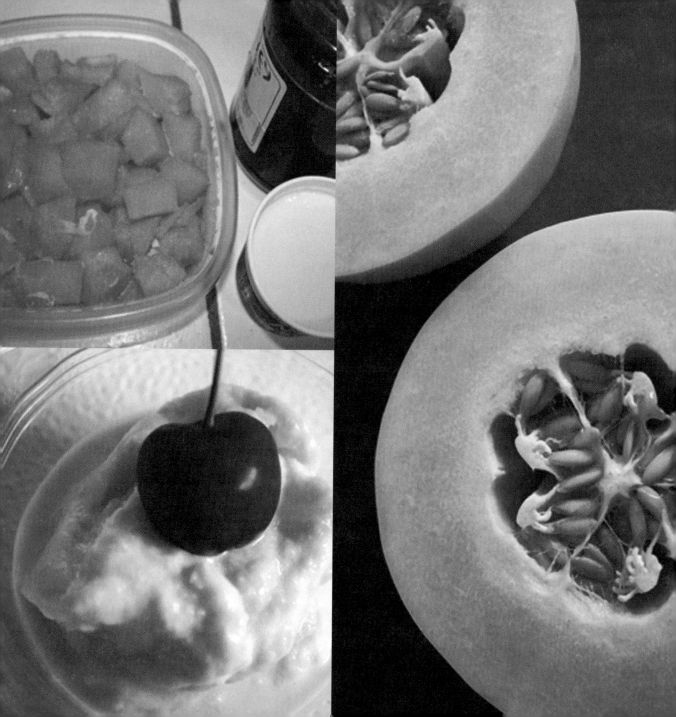

Instant Frozen Yogurt (Melon or Strawberry)

Makes about 3–5 cups

This recipe uses frozen fruit, which is blended with yogurt to achieve something close to soft-serve frozen yogurt. It works best with frozen chunks of ripe melon, almost as well with frozen strawberries, and reasonably well with slices of juicy peaches or plums. Most other fruits do not have the proper ratio of juice or the flavor to carry this dish. I sometimes freeze a small handful of banana slices and add this if the melon is not intensely flavored.

- 2–3 cups frozen fruit (start with two and add more if needed)
- ½ cup yogurt
- ½ cup sugar or substitute
- 1 tablespoon lemon juice

Do not thaw frozen fruit. Put all ingredients in blender and blend them together on a high setting. Scrape edges of the blender to make sure everything gets incorporated. If the frozen yogurt is too liquidy, then add a little more frozen fruit.

Chocolate-Chocolate Chip Frozen Yogurt

Makes about 3–4 cups

- 2 cups yogurt
- ½ cup cocoa powder (unsweetened)
- ½ cup sugar or substitute
- ½ teaspoon vanilla extract
- Handful or two of chocolate chips, milk or dark
- Optional: Replace ¼–½ cup of the yogurt with milk or cream to make it creamier and cut the sourness a bit

Put all ingredients, except for the chocolate chips, in a blender or food processor. Once they are well blended, add chocolate chips. If you like them whole, then stop blending. If you prefer them to be in smaller pieces and more incorporated, then blend on a pulse setting until they are the right size for you. Then follow directions in the Peach Ice Cream recipe (page 131) for freezing.

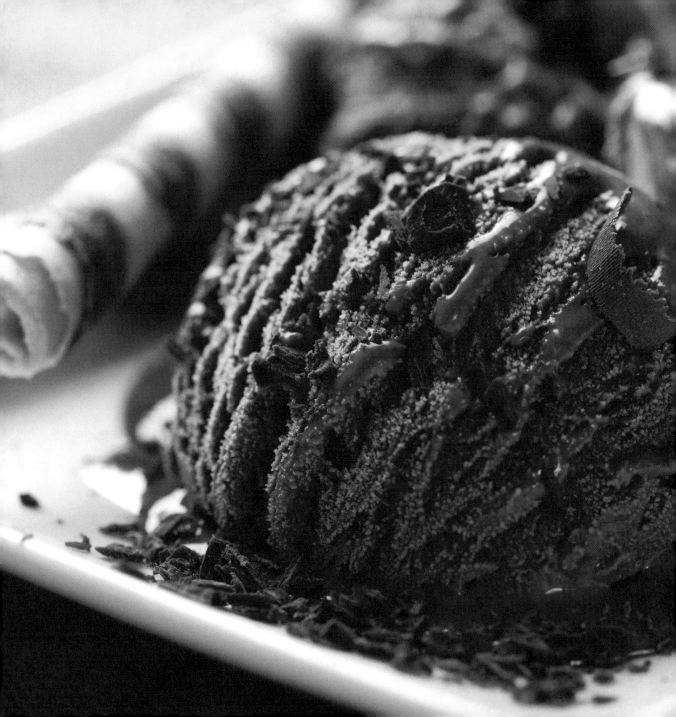

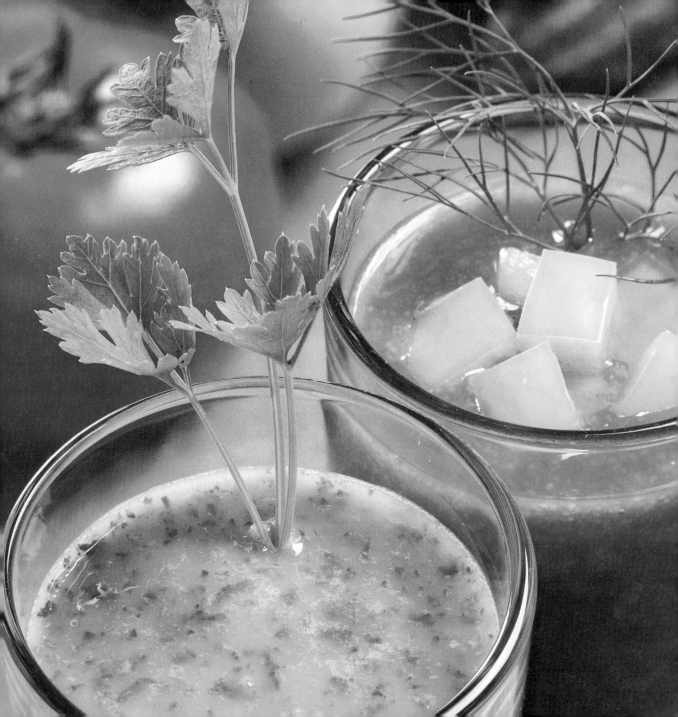

Chapter 18
Green Drinks and Healthy Energy Drinks

Green drinks and energy drinks are lumped into this chapter, but I will spend most of it covering energy drinks. Let's handle green drinks first, since I only have a few words to say about them. Basically, green drinks (whether the juice or smoothie variety) provide a great way to get some green foods and extra nutrition in your diet. You can combine green juice from spinach, kale, cucumber, celery, sunflower sprouts, and the like with something sweet (like apple juice) or savory (like tomato juice) if you wish. If you are really masochistic, you can combine green juice with some sour kombucha or water kefir!

Alternatively, and this is what most people do, you can create a green smoothie. Simply blend some green juice, green leaves (like baby spinach), or green juice powder with other ingredients. Green juice powders, available in health food stores, often contain spirulina or chlorella algae and/or powder from wheatgrass or other cereal grass juices, plus sometimes broccoli, kale, or spinach powder. Add some creamy yogurt or kefir, plus a banana and some apple juice, and aside from the color, you would never guess there is half a cup of spinach (or the green powder equivalent) in there. I have included several green drink recipes in this chapter, each of which essentially is a sweet or savory smoothie with green power as well as probiotic power. Drink one of these every morning and you can eat junk food the rest of the day!

Now, let's cover energy drinks. In theory, these are a great idea, but in practice, most commercially produced energy drinks do not provide healthy results. They are designed to give you a short-term fix with massive quantities of caffeine and sugar, combined with a questionable cocktail of herbs, vitamins, and amino acids such as guanine and taurine. Guanine is a stimulant derived from the guarana plant, which is high in caffeine, while the amino acid taurine serves to concentrate caffeine in the body.

Energy drinks have been blamed, rightly or wrongly, for a number of deaths. Many experts consider them to be unhealthy and perhaps dangerous to consume, particularly in combination with other active substances such as alcohol, tobacco, and more caffeine. Instead of consuming substances that squeeze the body for a short-term energy rush, why not make your own probiotic energy drink using safe and wholesome foods? These drinks can nourish the body and boost energy levels naturally. You can find many of the ingredients you need in your kitchen or cupboard.

Start with a base of kefir, water kefir, rejuvelac, or kombucha. Then add any of the ingredients below, each of which has been proven to have a positive effect on a person's energy. As always, if you are suffering from a particular medical condition, consult a qualified physician or natural health expert before making your own energy drinks or consuming any of the following substances that your body may not have encountered before (such as ginseng).

Cinnamon and Honey: Cinnamon has a warming flavor that adds a special touch to many foods and drinks. Honey, especially raw and unpasteurized honey with its enzymes intact, delivers a simple carbohydrate boost to your body. In a recent study, researchers found that cinnamon enhanced participants' brain functions and cognitive processing. Participants who smelled cinnamon or chewed cinnamon gum achieved better scores on a computer test of several different cognitive and memory functions. Separate research showed that taking half a teaspoon of honey sprinkled with cinnamon, around 3:00 p.m. each day, increases the body's vitality within a week at this time of the day when many people's body clocks are on a low ebb. It seems that a sprinkle of cinnamon is all you need to add to a homemade energy drink to get these benefits (and even the smell alone might do the job!). Large quantities of cinnamon can be toxic.

Citrus: Have you ever drank a glass of orange juice and felt more alert? When I stopped drinking coffee regularly many years ago, I often drank orange juice in the morning, and I swore it helped me wake up. It turns out I was not imagining this. Research has shown that both the smell of citrus and the acidity of the juice can awaken your body. Plus, it provides a great flavoring for any kefir, kombucha, natural soda, or energy drink. Try squeezing a little orange, lemon, lime, mandarin, or grapefruit juice into your drink.

Green Tea: Green tea can help increase your energy levels in several ways. First, since it contains some caffeine, you get a short-term boost. Typically, green tea contains much less caffeine than a cup of coffee, an energy drink, or a caffeinated soda. If you want the other benefits of green tea without the caffeine, you can opt for naturally decaffeinated green tea. To put green tea's caffeine level in perspective, consider the following list of the typical quantities of caffeine in these common sources. I think you'll find that green tea contains a smaller amount of caffeine than most alternatives:

- Green tea (8 oz): 25–40 mg of caffeine
- Black tea (8 oz): 15–60 mg
- Coca-Cola® (8 oz): 20–30 mg
- Monster™/Red Bull™/Rockstar™ Energy Drinks (8.0–8.4 oz): 80–92 mg
- 5-Hour Energy™ (2 oz): 207 mg
- Dark Chocolate (1.5 oz): 26 mg
- Milk chocolate (1.5 oz): 9 mg

The second way that green tea boosts your energy level is with a natural substance it contains called L-theanine, which has been shown to increase alertness without the jitters of caffeine. And third, EGCG is a powerful antioxidant in green tea that scrubs your body of free radicals. This should help you feel more energetic over time.

Ginseng: Thousands of years' worth of testing on humans has demonstrated ginseng's near-magical properties to the people of China, Korea, Japan, and beyond. More recently, Western studies have verified that panax ginseng (the most effective kind) really does boost energy. It may reach this result by improving blood flow to the brain. This is a natural increase that can be sustainable; it has none of the ups and downs associated with caffeine. Ginseng also is revered in Asia for its effect on sexual potency, which may also be related to the improved blood flow to the brain. Studies have proven that people who take ginseng before a test have better memory recognition and higher scores.

There are several kinds of ginseng, including American and Siberian, but panax ginseng (also known as red ginseng, Chinese red ginseng, or Korean ginseng) is the one that works best. I've tried a lot of herbs that are said to be good for one thing or another. Not one of them has ever worked on me the way panax ginseng does. If your energy is at a low ebb or you are feeling like you are getting a cold, drinking a strong cup of red ginseng tea might give you new life. It lifts me up a couple of levels on the energy meter and puts me back in a place where I feel like my body has the strength to fight off a pesky cold. If I felt like taking a nap before consuming ginseng, I often feel like running a mile or two after taking it (not always right away but within a few hours).

As for its potency powers? I will let you try it and see for yourself. Of course, make sure your physician approves if you have a medical condition or are on any medication, especially since I view ginseng as the strongest energy supplement in this chapter. Ginseng tea, extract, and powder generally are the best ways to add this to a probiotic beverage. It seems to deliver the most benefit at doses above 200 mg, but the label for the tea or extract you get may or may not include this information. Following the label directions is the best place to start, and from there you can adjust the amounts to your liking. If you cannot find ginseng locally at an Asian market or health food store, try conducting an online search for "red ginseng." It's worth every penny.

Mint: The smell and taste of mint can revive the senses. Try using a sprig of mint as an edible garnish or crush some mint and then soak it in water to make an extract for flavoring drinks. Another simple option is to brew some peppermint, spearmint, or pennyroyal tea, cool it, and add it to drinks.

Putting It All Together

There is a recipe below for a homemade probiotic energy drink, which includes all of these suggested enhancers. You do not need to include all of them; just use the ones you like and have available. If you need a big boost, though, I would suggest trying the ginseng, as it often has a stronger effect on energy levels than any other food. From citrus to cinnamon to mint tea, you may already have some of the others in your kitchen or cupboard.

Tea Bag Time Savers

If you do not have the time to brew up your own concoction, then here is a real time saver that just costs a few dollars. A number of tea companies, including Lipton®, Celestial Seasonings™, and Bigelow®/AriZona Iced Tea®, make and sell tea bags that include several energy-enhancing ingredients. All are available at stores that sell herbal teas or online. Lipton makes lemon ginseng green tea, Celestial Seasonings makes honey lemon ginseng green tea, and Bigelow (branded as AriZona) makes green tea with ginseng and honey. Rather than chasing down all the ingredients and measuring them, you could spend a few dollars for a box of twenty-five tea bags. Each time you needed an energy drink, you could heat a half cup or so of water, brew the tea bag in it until it cools a bit, then top off the cup with water kefir, rejuvelac, or kombucha. Add a little more honey, cinnamon, mint, or citrus squeeze if you wish. Wow, that was easy!

Here are the recipes for green drinks (which come first) and the energy drink (at the end of this chapter).

Secret Spinach Shake

Makes 4–6 cups

Sweet and dark fruit hide the two cups of baby spinach in this drink. You could use baby kale or other greens also. All fruit can be fresh or frozen.

- 1 ripe banana
- ½ cup orange juice
- 1 cup blueberries
- 1 cup pineapple
- 1 cup yogurt
- 2 cups baby spinach
- Honey or sugar, to taste

Place all ingredients in a blender. Blend, taste, adjust with additional honey or sugar, and serve.

Green Chocolate Chia

Makes 2–3 cups

This recipe uses chia seeds, which are incredibly nutritious and available at health food stores. If you prefer, you could substitute poppy seeds, hemp seed hearts, flax seeds, or ground flaxseed meal . . . or leave out the seeds if you just want the green chocolate! If you use chia, then presoak it as follows: put the chia seeds in a small cup, cover it with a little of the liquid you will use in the recipe (such as kombucha or kefir), and let the seeds soak for 5 minutes. Pour this into your blender, scraping in as many of the sticky seeds as you can get. Feel free to use as much spirulina, green powder, or spinach as you can handle.

- 1 cup chocolate ice cream or frozen yogurt (or 1 cup yogurt + 1 packet cocoa mix)
- 1–3 tablespoons chia seeds (presoaked as described above)
- 1–3 tablespoons (or more) spirulina or green juice powder or 1 cup baby spinach greens
- ¼ teaspoon vanilla extract
- 1 cup kombucha, kefir, or rejuvelac
- Optional: Handful of fresh mint leaves
- Garnish with a sprig of fresh mint

Place all ingredients in a blender. Blend, taste, adjust with additional honey or sugar, and serve.

Kale, Banana, and Pear Smoothie

Makes 2–3 cups

This recipe combines some very healthy greens with an overpowering quantity of sweet, custardy fruit (bananas and pears). Kale is easy to grow in the home garden and it is quite cold-hardy; we are able to grow it almost year-round. If you can only find tougher, mature kale leaves, then tear off the leafy parts and omit the stems. Another idea is to run your kale through a juicer first and just add the juice to this smoothie. Or you can substitute baby spinach leaves.

- 2 bananas
- 1 cup milk or CRASH alternative
- 2 ripe pears, peeled and cut
- 2 cups baby kale or baby spinach
- ½ cup yogurt or cottage cheese

Place all ingredients in a blender. Blend, taste, adjust with additional honey or sugar, and serve.

Beet and Green Kvass

Makes about 4–5 cups

Kvass is a traditional Russian drink, which usually is made with beets or dried rye bread. It is a sour-salty beverage. This recipe skips the rye bread, using only beets, greens, and celery. Due to these additional vegetables, it should be blended. You can culture this with yogurt whey, sauerkraut or natural pickle juice, or vegetable starter culture, or you can just skip the starter and rely on naturally present lactobacteria to ferment the vegetables a little more slowly (organic beets and celery have plenty of naturally present cultures). Like many fermented foods and drinks, kvass is an acquired taste. Those who do enjoy it often swear by its health benefits, some of them drinking kvass on a daily basis.

- 3 large beets, peeled and cut into cubes
- 1 quart water
- 1 stick celery, chopped
- Handful of baby spinach or baby kale
- 2 teaspoons whey/starter culture
- Optional: 1½–2 teaspoons sea salt
- Optional: 2 tablespoons ginger (chopped) or 1 clove garlic (crushed)

Place all ingredients in a blender, blend them together, and then move the drink to a container or jar. Cover it loosely and allow your beverage to ferment at room temperature for 3–5 days. Before drinking, add a little salt or sugar if you wish.

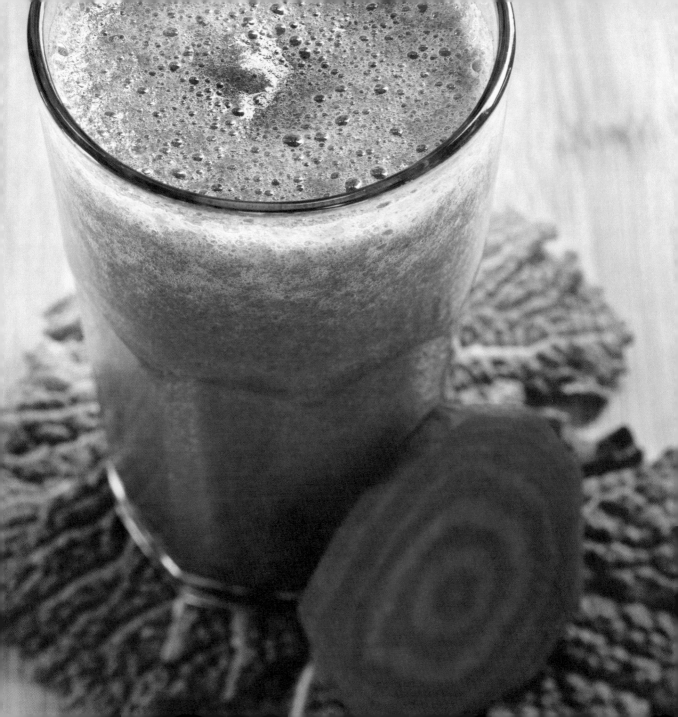

Savory Veggie Smoothie

This could be called V7, V9, or however many veggies you end up adding, though I don't wish to confuse it with a particular canned vegetable juice. You can make this as salty or spicy as you want by adding salt and jalapeno pepper. For an extra probiotic kick, throw in a little sauerkraut or natural pickles if you have some! If this smoothie is too fibrous for you, then another option is to run these veggies through a juicer and just add their juice to the blender along with the other ingredients.

- 1 cup tomato juice
- ½ cup carrot juice
- ½ cup kombucha, water kefir, or rejuvelac
- ½ cucumber, peeled
- 1 small celery stalk
- ¼ cup bell pepper
- ½ cup baby spinach or baby kale greens
- 1 small clove of garlic (crushed) or small handful of fresh chives
- 1 teaspoon lemon or lime juice
- Salt, black pepper, and cayenne pepper, to taste

- Optional: ½ jalapeno pepper
- Optional: ¼ cup sauerkraut or natural pickles

Place all ingredients in a blender. Blend, taste, adjust with additional honey or sugar, and serve.

Carrot Seaweed Green Smoothie

Makes about 2 cups

You can buy dried seaweed in Asian and health food stores. Look for kelp (kombu), though most other kinds will work fine. Try incorporating a few different kinds of seaweed to create a diverse range of nutrition and taste. To rehydrate the seaweed, soak it in water for at least 2 hours or until it is soft. The seaweed will still be firm, but moist throughout.

- ½ cup dried seaweed (soaked in water for at least 2 hours or until tender)
- 1–1½ cups carrot juice
- ½ cup kombucha, water kefir, or rejuvelac
- ¼ inch fresh ginger, peeled and chopped
- Optional: 1 banana, if you want to go the sweeter route

Healthy Energy Drink

Makes about 2 cups

- 1 cup water, boiled
- 200 milligrams panax ginseng (extract or powder) *or* 1 panax ginseng tea bag (100–500 milligram strength)
- 1 teaspoon dried green tea leaves *or* 1 green tea bag
- Squeeze of lemon, lime, grapefruit, or orange
- 1 cup kombucha, water kefir, or cider
- Honey or sugar, to taste

Pour water (slightly below boiling temperature) over ginseng and green tea. Let steep for 3 minutes. Remove tea bags or pour tea liquid into another cup or container, straining out the tea leaves if needed. Then let the tea sit or place in the refrigerator until it cools to below 100°F. Mix in honey or sugar if you wish. Then combine with other ingredients. Garnish with a sprig of mint or a slice of citrus.

Grapefruit Mint Energy Drink

Makes 2–3 cups

- 2 cups kombucha or water kefir
- Juice of 1 grapefruit
- ¼ cup Mint Soda Syrup (see chapter on making sodas for recipe)

Combine all ingredients and serve. Garnish with fresh mint.

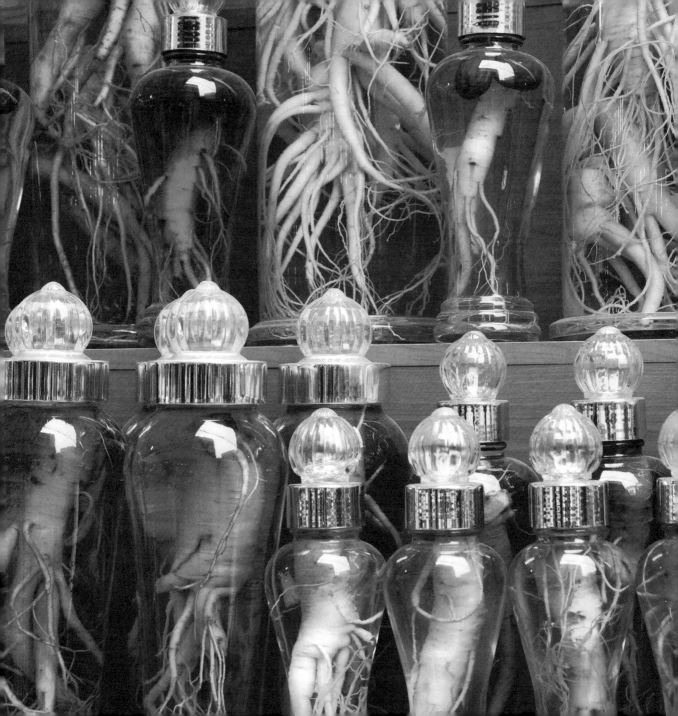

Mandarin Orange Spice Energy Drink

- 2 cups natural cider
- Juice of 3–4 mandarin oranges or tangerines
- Pinch of cinnamon
- Thin slice of ginger (peeled) *or* pinch of powdered ginger
- Optional: Pinch of allspice or 1 clove

Combine orange juice with spices. If you have time, put this in the refrigerator and let it sit for a few minutes or hours. Then combine with cider.

Appendix
Resources

Most equipment and food supplies in this book can be found locally. Many health food stores or home-brewing supply stores stock the equipment you will need to make cheese, ciders, and sodas. If you need an odd vegetable or spice, then try an ethnic grocery store. For example, if you want to use authentic Korean chili pepper powder, then try an Asian market. If you would like to find some Moroccan spice, then try a Middle Eastern or North African store.

But assuming you cannot find what you need locally, here are some good online resources.

Herbs and Spices

Frontier Co-op, www.frontiercoop.com
Starwest Botanicals, www.starwest-botanicals.com
Zamouri Spices, www.zamourispices.com
Latin Merchant, www.latinmerchant.com
Korean Ginseng Shop, www.kgcus.com
In the UK: The Asian Cookshop, www.theasiancookshop.co.uk
And everything else seems to be available at: www.amazon.com

Cheese Supplies

New England Cheesemaking Supply, www.cheesemaking.com
The Cheesemaker (Wisconsin), www.thecheesemaker.com
Midwest Supplies, www.midwestsupplies.com

Sources of Kefir, Kombucha, and Other Cultures

Cultures for Health, www.culturesforhealth.com
Royal Kombucha, www.royalkombucha.com
Kombucha Brooklyn, www.kombuchabrooklyn.com
Body Ecology, www.bodyecology.com
Yemoos (has Ginger Beer Plant and others), www.yemoos.com
If you're brave enough: eBay, www.ebay.com

Soda, Cider, Pickling, and Crock Supplies

Leener's, www.leeners.com
Northwest Cider Supply, www.northwestcidersupply.com
World Market (has clamp-top soda bottles), www.worldmarket.com
Pickl-It, www.pickl-it.com
Fermenta Caps, www.fermentacaps.com
Crate and Barrel (carries Le Parfait canning jars), www.crateandbarrel.com
Mountain Feed and Farm Supply (great selection of fermenting crocks),
    www.mountainfeed.com

Recipe Index

The HEALTHY probiotic Diet

METRIC AND IMPERIAL CONVERSIONS

(These conversions are rounded for convenience)

Ingredient	Cups/Tablespoons/ Teaspoons	Ounces	Grams/Milliliters
Fruits or veggies, chopped	1 cup	5 to 7 ounces	145 to 200 grams
Honey or maple syrup	1 tablespoon	.75 ounce	20 grams
Liquids: cream, milk, water, or juice	1 cup	8 fluid ounces	240 milliliters
Spices: cinnamon, cloves, ginger, or nutmeg (ground)	1 teaspoon	0.2 ounce	5 milliliters
Sugar, brown, firmly packed	1 cup	7 ounces	200 grams
Sugar, white	1 cup/1 tablespoon	7 ounces/0.5 ounce	200 grams/12.5 grams
Vanilla extract	1 teaspoon	0.2 ounce	4 grams

OVEN TEMPERATURES

Fahrenheit	Celcius	Gas Mark
225°	110°	¼
250°	120°	½
275°	140°	1
300°	150°	2
325°	160°	3
350°	180°	4
375°	190°	5
400°	200°	6
425°	220°	7
450°	230°	8

Notes

Notes

Notes

Notes

Notes

Notes

Notes